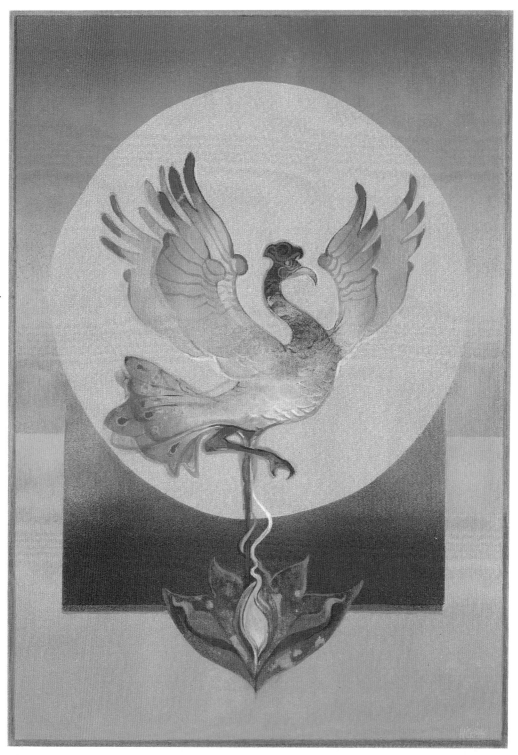

The Phoenix Stands on One Leg.

T'AI-CHI
Spirit and Essence

A New Vision of a Healing Process

BEVERLEY MILNE

*An introduction to the nature, form
and spirit of a masterpiece*

*A Way of Life for those
on the Spiritual Path and all
sincere seekers*

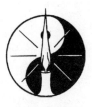

— Published by —
The Healing School of T'ai-Chi
Melbourne, Australia

First Edition (London)   July 1979

Second Edition (Revised and Enlarged)   October 1994

National Library of Australia card number and

ISBN 0 646 19580 8

Typesetting and design by Robert John, MAS & Associates, Melbourne

Printed and bound in Australia by McPherson's Printing Group

ABOUT THE AUTHOR

Beverley Milne was born in Adelaide, and lived in London for 28 years. Originally an art teacher, then an opera singer, she has from 1971 served as an inner teacher, healer and writer. She created The School of T'ai-chi Ch'uan Centre for Healing in London over 20 years, and was a leading communicator of this art in the U.K.

In addition to T'ai-chi, she has over the last 20 years given a variety of workshops in spiritual science, meditation, healing and therapy, providing a rounded spiritual education for her T'ai-chi students and many others. T'ai-chi Teaching and Intuitive Foot Massage are both Certificate courses. She is a Full Member of the International Association for Colour Therapy (MIACT).

Having given workshops, ABC talks and interviews in Australia since 1980, she became a Melbourne resident in 1990 and established The Healing School of T'ai-Chi. With her wide background in creative arts, spiritual science and Eastern philosophy, T'ai-chi, "I Ching" and healing, Beverley found her own individuality as a creative medium through teaching and lecturing, counselling and writing.

Beverley Milne's inner teaching is not drawn from any one spiritual source. She projects her own reality, drawing constantly from personal experience, her own soul resources and spiritual guidance. She acknowledges her foundation studies in esoteric training and traditions, and all who have inspired her. Her sole object is to seek and project Truth, Beauty and Harmony.

CONTENTS

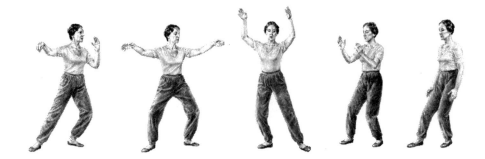

Part II –
THE T'AI-CHI EXPERIENCE:
COLOUR AND CLAIRVOYANT RESEARCH

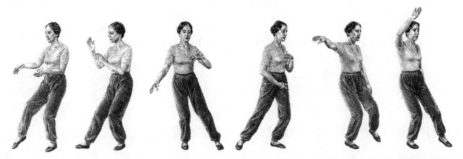

Reproduced with permission from Readers' Digest (Aust.) Pty. Ltd. from the book *Family Guide to Alternative Medicine*

Part III –
STUDENTS' EXPERIENCES
AND FURTHER OBSERVATIONS

APPENDICES

FOREWORD

The aim of this introductory book is to revive and shed new light on the true essence and spirit of T'ai-chi Ch'uan. My thoughts herein are naturally the expression of personal feeling, to communicate a perspective of identification and communion with the One Life, and with the rhythms and harmonies of Nature, its colour and its music. This perspective receives as yet little projection, either in teaching or in print, but its meaning and validity will become increasingly apparent as we move forward into the new Age of the brotherhood of humanity.

I feel also a concern to help redirect the energies of the modern world's insatiable enthusiasm for 'doing' and 'attaining' – even within the very art which is designed to teach a greater wisdom. Much of the genius and healing nature of T'ai-chi, and the mental, emotional and spiritual significance of movement itself has yet to be recognized, while too much emphasis continues to be laid on old Chinese cultural realities or modern indulgences. In the light of greater knowledge, this universal art is developing and will continue to develop, and outdated traditionalism or current superficialities will be transcended by time and enlightenment.

By the full meaning of its name, T'ai-chi embraces the interdependence of all aspects of Nature and her processes – visible and invisible, positive and negative, physical and spiritual. This is not only co-ordination of the body-mind, or even the perception, balancing and integration of all physical/temporal energies – body, etheric, emotional and conscious mental – admittedly a major task; it is not to do with defending the self, but *letting go* of the personality ego through self-discipline and realization. The 'supreme ultimate' of T'ai-chi is expansion of consciousness, the linking via the bridge of the mind with the higher Spiritual Self, and the permeation and transmutation onto a higher arc of being of the whole personality by the unique Soul Individuality. Hence the body, which is the link between inner Self and objective world, must be directed by the mind as a living vehicle of experience and the channel of creative expression.

My interests are in the 'wholemaking' process. Healing by touch, aura, massage, diet, thought projection, manipulation etc. are most valuable, and essential at given times, but they are external and therefore relatively temporary. The real focus must be to reach into the mind and inspire the soul – to adjust the view of self and outlook on life, thus raising the vibration from the *inside*. In all my work therefore, particularly through T'ai-chi, and with Meditation, Spiritual Counselling, Intuitive Foot Massage, Colour Healing etc., my approach is through spiritual teaching, meditation and general instruction in natural law and natural therapeutics: To 'heal' the body without approaching reason, feeling and the soul is superficial and a waste of time.

It is my joy that T'ai-chi Ch'uan is a masterly embodiment of spiritual teaching and natural therapeutics. Relaxation and stability on all levels, good body alignment and breathing, or any of the benefits listed at the end of this book, can only be the outward reflections of inner harmonies. In becoming receptive and adaptable in all situations, and sensitive to experience at all levels, one has the possibility of finding the true core of life in all aspects of one's own Individuality.

— Beverley Milne, 1979
— Revised expanded edition, 1994

INTRODUCTION
The Heritage of Yang Style

The root and style of T'ai-chi Ch'uan which I practice and teach is known as Yang.

T'ai-chi in the modern Western world generally stems from the teaching and practice of the style of Yang Lu-chan, who was given permission to teach it publicly in Beijing in c.1850. (see Chapter 7). In being handed down through the many generations which have followed, there have evolved other styles (especially in the U.S.A.), some of them quite good, but many of them very self-indulgent and of little real therapeutic value – certainly as compared with the authentic art form. This latter situation occurs usually where there is more enthusiasm than genuine knowledge of either philosophy or therapeutics. Since the T'ai-chi is a living art, and its practitioners human and of varying abilities and perception, it is inevitable that in some hands there will be a loss of technique and understanding, in other hands a fairly faithful maintaining of tradition or teaching, and in a few hands the re-alignment with knowledge and root principles, possibly creative development.

The Form Style inherited by myself and taught in The Healing School of T'ai-Chi in Melbourne (and The School of T'ai-chi Ch'uan Centre for Healing, London, founded by me) is classical Yang, as learnt and passed down through his grandson Yang Cheng-fu to Choy Hawk-peng (in Hong Kong), and his son Choy Kam-man, and thence via Gerda Geddes (in London) to myself. Although there were clearly a few structural errors in the form (most of which have been re-aligned), the form taught in this School is acknowledged to be fairly pure and refined. In being very subtle, it is a very beautiful form. Indeed I am constantly endeavouring to refine its energies and expression. The inherent allegory of the T'ai-chi cycle, recognized by my predecessor, inspired me to develop this area of the teaching with its practical and inspirational applications as a very important communication within our present-day material culture. It is passed on as an essential part of my Teacher Training Programme.

Otherwise, the philosophical, spiritual, symbolic and therapeutic perception and projection is my own reality, born of my own studies and experience in Eastern and Western philosophy, spiritual science, physiology, natural medicine and therapies. I have never been inclined to follow any particular 'master' in the external sense, Chinese or otherwise, but relied upon my own perceptions of intuition, clairvoyance, practical and spiritual knowledge, and in many instances – common sense. My prior training and experience in teaching, art, drama, music and theatre are of immeasurable value in my appreciation and communication of the art.

Certainly all resources must be blended into an integrated whole, and not least do I listen to the Chinese in my soul.

— Beverley Milne, 1994

PART I

T'AI-CHI
Spirit & *Essence*

CHAPTER 1
Origins

T'ai-chi Ch'uan is a callisthenic fine art, born of inspiration in the 11th Century, and its present movement form dating from about the 14th Century A.D. Its origins and roots are in Chinese history and culture, more particularly in its philosophy (mainly Taoist, Ch'an, and in more recent centuries Buddhist, with Confucian influences), 'yogic' breathing techniques, alchemical investigation and seermanship (clairvoyance), medical therapies and self-defence exercises. A cultural masterpiece developed in the monasteries, the true art was until the mid 19th Century virtually an esoteric school available only within the monasteries and temple schools, and certain families of culture.

Exercising – for health or self-defence, has always been a traditional part of Chinese culture. Earliest exercises for general health and strength dating from thousands of years ago recognized four factors which have together formed the basis of Chinese exercises and medicine:

1. Man is a microcosmic reflection of Macrocosmic Law.

2. All life is movement and change within Unity.

3. The human organism is designed to function as an integrated whole.

4. Prevention is better than cure.

These are the premises upon which Chinese acupuncture, herbal medicine, therapeutic and callisthenic exercises such as T'ai-chi Ch'uan, and self-defence techniques have been built.

The observation that mind and body are intimately linked and that the mind directly affects the body, made it obvious that anxiety etc., causing tension, causes dis-ease or sickness by interfering with breathing, circulation and general body functioning. An active but peaceful mind was recognized as necessary to health and balanced personality as an efficient body.

To maintain a state of naturalness and flow in all aspects of the personality therefore, therapeutic exercises were developed imitating bird and animal movements and sounds owing to their unselfconscious naturalness, which also formed the basis of their dances. About the beginning of the Christian era, these natural movements were formulated into exercises called the Five Animals Frolics, and co-ordinated breathing with movement. Hua T'o, a noted surgeon of the 3rd Century A.D. devised a therapeutic system of exercises largely derived from them, and is reputed to have said:

> *The ancients practised the bear's neck, the fowl's twist, swaying the body, and moving the joints to prevent old age and achieve longevity. I have a system of exercises called the Frolics of the Five Animals ... which are the tiger, the deer, the bear, the monkey and the bird. It removes disease, strengthens the legs, and ensures good health.* He also said, *The used doorstep never rots.*

An excellent example of these available today are the Five Animals Movements, as offered by The Healing School of T'ai-Chi (see Appendix B). Hua T'o realized that relaxation was necessary for health, and could not be attained by straining: the complete absorption seen in animals in their activities was the key reflecting the necessary stillness of mind and mental focus. He understood that "exercises must not be done to the point of exhaustion". The balanced containing and controlling of energy thus became the guiding principle in all exercise systems – therapeutic, callisthenic and self-defence, as it had been in early Taoist monasteries.

Since 6th – 5th Centuries B.C., such exercises had been evolved by the Quietists and later Taoist nature mystics. Taoists aimed to attain complete Union with Tao – the unnameable Essence of All Being, via practices to attain inner stillness, finer mental focus, harmony and flowing with the processes of life. Body movements were co-ordinated with 'yogic' breathing exercises[1], with their growing knowledge of subtle (esoteric) anatomy, and the balancing of the movements of energies which they called *ch'i* (= *ki* or *prana*). Within this of course was naturally the influence of exercises of unarmed combat, the heritage of all cultured Chinese.

By the early centuries of the Christian era, these exercises became known as *kung-fu*, workout exercises which one could practice to help oneself. They were evolved largely by physicians (who were almost always of the Taoist belief), and taught in little schools attached to their practices, for their chief work was preventive medicine. They were not paid if those under their care became ill. In time, these exercises became the expression of creation myths, in which the people could identify with the processes of nature and creation, and through them find release.

Although still very influenced by the original Taoist principles – the acceptance of natural cyclic movements and flow in all nature, and their pure (spiritual) alchemical *yogas* for attaining spiritual immortality (Union with Tao), exercises were by the early Christian era increasingly and most valuably influenced by *degenerate* alchemy: Having long attempted to defy natural law in seeking physical immortality, the more physically-oriented Taoist monks had at last resigned themselves to its impossibility, and shifted their attention to the attainment of long life.

---

[1] See "Taoism, The Mystical Way of Lao Tzu", by Beverley Milne.

The function and use of the body and subtle energies then became subject to much finer scrutiny, especially in the monasteries and temple schools. Monks were concerned both to preserve and to improve the quality of life, and secondarily to develop some skills of self-defence without the use of weapons – which they weren't permitted to carry. *Kung-fu* were gradually refined and lengthened to require the finer balancing of energies necessary for *endurance*. Always involving continuity and flow of movement, they were aided considerably by the observations of energy movements by enlightened seers (clairvoyants), together with the experience of physicians, athletes and self-defence experts, especially during the period of Taoist revival of the 2nd and 3rd Centuries.

In this way, *ch'uan* exercises were evolved. *Ch'uan* means literally 'fist', which is a nucleus or focus of energy and therefore a symbol of energy containment. They were designed for the controlling of one's temporal nature – the mastery of mind, emotion and body, and were of self-defence as well as of therapeutic value.

Suggestions for further reading:

- Taoism, the Way of the Mystic – J.C. Cooper (Aquarian Press)
- Yin and Yang – J.C. Cooper (Aquarian Press)
- The Secret and Sublime –Taoist Mysteries & Magic – John Blofeld (Routledge K.P.)
- The Way of Life According to Lao Tzu (Tao Tê Ching) – trans. Witter Bynner
- Chuang Tzu – translated by Herbert Giles (or other)
- The Secret of the Golden Flower – trans. Richard Wilhelm (Penguin Arkana)

CHAPTER 2
The Birth of T'ai-chi Ch'uan

Chang San-feng

In the 11th Century A.D., within an age of great movement and development in Chinese thought (the Sung Dynasty), a new *ch'uan* was born through the spiritual inspiration of a young nobleman called Chang San-feng.

A highly sensitive, spiritually and psychically awakened soul, Chang was deeply disturbed by the aggressive nature of the Shaolin martial training in which he was by birth obliged to engage. Deserting the army, he became a hermit for some twelve years, cautiously re-emerging inspired to reform exercising along soul and spiritual lines of harmony, love and brotherhood. Initially he trained army men in the way of compassion. Later he drew other devoted disciples and developed a more subtle *ch'uan* – a long *kung-fu* eventually of some 20 minutes duration. This was built around the principles of soft yielding and flowing, and an awareness of the evolutionary processes of man within the Universe. It marked the beginnings of distinctly 'intrinsic' or internal mystical exercising, embracing the whole nature of man. (Other developments of 'intrinsic' exercising are Pa Kua and Hsing I, but these are both martial arts, not holistic therapies.)

Although high born and well educated, and with the clairvoyant gifts of the spirit, Chang did not have the more detailed esoteric knowledge of the Taoist monks and seers who became the heirs to his work. He was an inspired mystic, around whom many fantasies and stories have inevitably developed.

In the following centuries, the work was taken up and evolved in Taoist and later Buddhist monasteries and temple schools as an 'intrinsic' (internal) therapeutic and healing art, and it became in their hands more specifically built around the philosophy and symbolism of T'ai-chi which was developed in the 12th Century. In aiming for mastery and integration of the whole Self, it acquired by the 15th Century the name T'ai-chi Ch'uan. It was subsequently developed by Buddhist monks increasingly as a highly sophisticated healing process, art expression and creation mime play, building upon elements which had been inherent in exercising for thousands of years.

The martial associations (although not entirely the martial terminology) from which the art was partly derived had long since filtered away, since the principles of yielding and transmuting the personality to the Spirit were incompatible with defending the self. For people in the modern world endeavouring to follow a spiritual Path, self-defence is irrelevant and superfluous: For the spiritualized man who flows with life, self-defence does not exist.

The Meaning of T'ai-chi

As an early Chinese concept dating back thousands of years, *t'ai-chi* originally meant 'ridgepole' (i.e. central support or mainstay), philosophically (or cosmologically) the link or One-ness of Life bridging Heaven and Earth. It was symbolically represented by the *line*: | or –.

During the flowering of thought in the Sung Dynasty however (c. 10th – 12th Centuries A.D.), T'ai-chi came to mean more specifically the Great or Supreme Ultimate or Supreme Limit – the underlying Unity which is all Creation. It is the Macrocosm embracing within itself the equilibrium of constant cyclic and sequent movements of change which are the characteristic expression of Universal Law: manifestation. These movements ebb and flow between the complementary polarities of (to the Chinese) Yin and Yang (Earth and Heaven) – the yielding and the firm, dark and light, receptive and creative, negative and positive, subjective and objective, below and above etc. The Master Lao Tzu says in the "Tao Tê Ching", the principle Taoist classic accredited to him:

> *By the blending of the breath*
> *From the sun and the shade,*
> *Equilibrium comes to the world."*
>
> (Ch. 42. Blakney trans.)

In literature these rhythmic, cyclic processes of natural law are embodied in the "I Ching" (pronounced Ye Jing), the ancient Book of Changes (Transformations); in movement they are embodied in the living, poetic beauty of T'ai-chi Ch'uan. For this reason, the study of "I Ching" may naturally if not essentially accompany the study of T'ai-chi.[1]

The diagram which was adopted as the T'ai-chi symbol was a very ancient one. The polar forces therein expressed had become termed Yin and Yang during the 3rd Century B.C.[2], and it is still often called the Yin-Yang Diagram. The meaning of "T'ai-chi T'u" (T'ai-chi Diagram) is of course as central practically, philosophically and spiritually to T'ai-chi Ch'uan as it is to the "I Ching". Spiritually understood, the movement of the polar energies activated by the *ch'i* is clockwise on the objective level of the diagram (anticlockwise in the inherent subjective level), with the light Yang force ascending and the dark Yin force sinking according to their essential natures. See the box page following.

T'ai-chi Ch'uan

T'ai-chi (macrocosm) being the underlying Unity of all life, the art of T'ai-chi

───────────────────────────────────

[1] See "Consulting the *I Ching*", by Beverley Milne.

[2] See "A Survey of Chinese Thought", by Beverley Milne, p.13.

T'ai-chi
(The Macrocosm)

Symbol of Eternal Law in Manifestation

the wavelike flow of movment, stirred by *ch'i* (subtle energy)

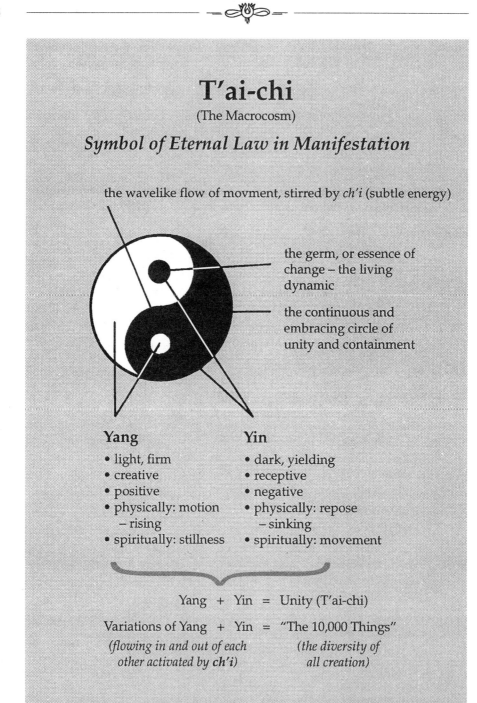

the germ, or essence of change – the living dynamic

the continuous and embracing circle of unity and containment

Yang
- light, firm
- creative
- positive
- physically: motion
  – rising
- spiritually: stillness

Yin
- dark, yielding
- receptive
- negative
- physically: repose
  – sinking
- spiritually: movement

Yang + Yin = Unity (T'ai-chi)

Variations of Yang + Yin = "The 10,000 Things"

*(flowing in and out of each   (the diversity of
other activated by **ch'i**)   all creation)*

Tao is universal law, and T'ai-chi is its manifestation

Ch'uan (microcosm) embraces much more than those *denser* aspects of life which are relatively tangible and objective. It involves not only the balancing of mental, emotional and physical energies – the elements of the personality subject to the processes of change, symbolically called the Tiger in T'ai-chi Ch'uan.

The art aims for the integration and therefore complete mastery of the *whole Individuality* – the self-realized, spiritualized human being. Such mastery requires the balancing of *all* energies – the physical with the spiritual, the personality (Tiger) with the Spirit, through the alignment of energies and opening of the higher spiritual faculties of Inspiration, Intuition and Spiritual Will. This is the process of self-realization.

Such is the object of the mature inner school of T'ai-chi Ch'uan. Essential aspects of training (certainly in my Schools) therefore include body alignment and dynamics, experience and study of energy movements – including discussion and awareness of dietary and sexual balance, meditation and breathing (including imagery and colour for release and healing), symbolism and philosophy of change, and spiritual science. *All aspects must be related to modern life*, for by this we may understand our essential nature as a microcosm within the Macrocosm. Wholeness *essentially* implies the inclusion of the higher spiritual principles, and the *degree* of wholeness attained will be reflected outwardly in our health at all levels of expression. It will be reflected in relating harmoniously and in awareness, not only with family and friends, but with the whole environment of all kingdoms of nature, seen and unseen.

Realization

The integrative process is directed by the mind, which must become subject to the detached application of the Spiritual Will: Being the bridge between the physical and the spiritual, in due course of development the mind masters the body, and thus opens the way beyond the reasoning intellect into the higher intuitive mind to become the servant of the Spirit. In T'ai-chi Ch'uan this is attained through the growing understanding, relaxation, focus and discipline of the Tiger – the temporal and changeable aspects of man's personality, into a balanced alignment with a common centre of gravity. Through this alignment of energies and the creation of 'inner space', the higher Spiritual energies can descend, permeate and thus *transmute*. This is the 'ultimate' of T'ai-chi Ch'uan – to refine or raise the vibrations of *every* aspect of the individual, so aiding his spiritual evolution. It is the process of emptying the self, *enabling the personality to become the crucible of Spiritual expression.*

The movement towards the realization of T'ai-chi, i.e. the unity in awareness, is therefore our conscious endeavour towards balance and harmony within ourselves and with our environment on every level of being. In practical terms, this means not only movement towards attaining *inward* harmony, but the recognition that each of us is required in due course *to realize and express outwardly our own unique individuality.* This requires in fact many lifetimes to achieve. Very few people in our world have attained to this stage, most of us yet being reflections of parental, environmental and cultural patterns, but it is for us all the pre-requisite during the earth-life for our eventual release and Union with Tao, union with the Godhead or Divine Source. The idea that we must 'lose' our identity in the T'ai-chi, Tao, Nirvana etc. is a naïve misconception, for we cannot lose what we have yet to find: it is to aim for the stars when we must first reach the ceiling of our Earth (and higher) experience. Even when we *do* attain enlightenment it is relative to the Earth experience, not absolute, and we will feel an inner compulsion (universal Love) to help others on the Path.

What we *do* have to lose in this life is the *divisive nature* of the self-centred ego of the personality. This requires us through knowledge and experience to *understand* that ego-nature, and to so apply the Spiritual Will (not self-will) to discipline the ego into balanced co-operation with the Spirit. This is the way of realization towards the expression of unique Individuality. In short, our lives should gradually pertain more to the nature of Tao (pure Being) – or initially T'ai-chi (Unity), and less to the nature of separateness and self-centredness; i.e. to identify with the One. It is the realizing of our true nature, the spiritual potential which has been present within all along, but the light of which has long been obscured by the selfish whims of the personality. T'ai-chi Ch'uan is not a passport to such spirituality; it is a framework through which the soul can grow in balance.

Unfortunately, but owing to human nature inevitably, the art of T'ai-chi Ch'uan has in recent centuries been misunderstood by the spiritually immature. Its superior and masterly techniques of subtlety being discovered by the Chinese nobility and the army, the art was sought and seized upon for application outside the monasteries, and degenerated into self-defence associations which it had long since advanced beyond. Other techniques using sticks and swords (now often considered traditional) were eventually developed. Although excellent physical/mental exercises with rooting in philosophy and laws of dynamics, and fascinating – often beautiful to watch, they are, in being physically rather than spiritually oriented (in spite of the aura which people sometimes project around them), alien to the inner philosophy and spirit of T'ai-chi.

It is unfortunate that the self-defence arts have remained under the same name as the integrative art of healing. The only sword in the mature study of T'ai-chi Ch'uan is metaphoric and symbolic – the two-edged Sword of Truth. The Pushing Hands exercise however, a rhythmic practice to develop fine sensing between two people, is a valuable extension to the main long solo form. Today of course, as in earlier days, there are teachers who like myself are continuing to develop other newer and sometimes better exercises and practices. Providing one knows and applies the principles correctly, there is no reason to be hidebound by traditional practices, but rather to evolve further according to the needs and insights of the Age.

CHAPTER 3
The Nature of the Forms

Accepting Limitation

In design and purpose, T'ai-chi Ch'uan is a microcosmic reflection and embodiment of the framework of Natural Law (Tao) and the processes of change. The essential nature of this Law and the limitations of the phenomenal world we must understand, accept and work within. Attempts to resist, ignore or override these limitations, whether consciously or unconsciously, incur tension, disharmony and ultimately disease.

T'ai-chi is a perfect vehicle for teaching the law of *karma* – that we reap what we sow, the law of return and rebound. Forms can be taught not only as movement between polarities, but the *principle explained*, illustrated and understood by directly relating it to the student's personal experience: to overreach here is to sacrifice there; to underplay now will require compensation later etc. Lao Tzu said "To grasp is to lose", and "The biggest problem in the world could have been solved when it was small". A microcosm where we can come to terms with the nature and limitations of life, T'ai-chi shows the necessity of accepting responsibility for our own actions – in thought and feeling, as well as body. What I call 'instant *karma*' is demonstrated in every class, and the opportunity presented to explain how an effect is tied to a cause, rather than merely saying "that's not right" or "it's like this".

T'ai-chi is outwardly a set framework of forms which the student accepts and does not in any way alter to suit himself, any more than he can alter his own bone structure. It is a mirror of the order of life: whatever the ease or difficulty, all situations must be faced, accepted and worked through until all is in harmony. There is no avoidance of the issue, only possibly a deferment until one is prepared for it. Harmony found within the movements will be a reflection of the harmony acquired in the self, and is the key to fuller relationships in the objective world. The forms (or form – for there is in essence only One) are therefore a vehicle, a sounding-board for a life-long growing process of experience, discovery and realization, its discipline teaching self-analysis in a quiet, objective and constructive way. For such reasons, T'ai-chi is a valuable key in the restoration of personal and social sanity in the modern civilized world!

In aiming for subtlety and inner stillness, not physical strength – 'to be' rather than 'to do', the movement exercises and enables the individual to explore all aspects of himself concurrently without any strain, rush or fatigue, and to co-ordinate mind, feelings, body, breath and spirit into balanced harmony. There are no postures or stretching, for everything finds its naturalness in alignment and flow within the framework. If the forms are taught *well* with clarity and insight, the student experiences and realizes them as simply a refined 'condensation' of much larger, more sweeping rhythms – a microcosmic expression of Macrocosmic design. In approaching them in the right way of naturalness, there is no feeling of limitation or restriction, no sense of repression, but rather the awakening to the joy of *simplicity, space and beauty of line* in movement and feeling.

Physical Structure

The movements of T'ai-chi consist of the shifting of weight and energies between opposite polarities in space, with the mind remaining in tranquillity the coordinating factor and overseer. The body is loosely 'weighted' through the base of the spine, and rooted in the legs and feet through the precision of well-spread, cat-like foot placement. Lao Tzu says "One may move so well that a footprint never shows."[1] The movement rides easily along the smooth and constant shifting of weight through bended legs like the pouring of liquid, as if suspended through the crown of the head, the circular gestures of arms and upper body linked fluidly (freed from tension) via the free-flowing waist. As Lao Tzu says

> Gravity is the root of grace,
> The mainstay of all speed.

and

> Always the low carry the high
> On a root for growing by.[2]

So the whole organism 'breathes' with Heaven and Earth through head and feet. There is no waste, no strain, and no jar.

Structurally, the foot-stepping through the 8 basic directions in the 2-dimensional square of the floor plan– the square being the symbol of the Earth and earth-nature, provides the basic body rooting, the physical-psychological certainty and security to which one yields. This rooting makes possible the upper body's light and easy circular carriage of curving and spiralling through the 3-dimensions of space, the circle being the symbol of Heaven, completeness, unity and continuity. Flowing alternations between polarities (between Yin and Yang) are thus facilitated in every conceivable way as the T'ai-chi-style Way of experience and expression– between firm and yielding, masculine and feminine, up and down, in and out and so on.

---

[1] "The Way of Life According to Lao Tzu", ch.27, Bynner trans.

[2] Ibid., ch's.26, 29.

Thus T'ai-chi Ch'uan works even structurally with the harmonizing of the circle and the square, Heaven and Earth, Yang and Yin. Circular, spirallic movement is specifically recognized and cultivated in this art, even down to the tiniest movements in obscure joints, but is of course inevitable, since there are no straight lines in the universe. See the diagrams on page 14.

The 8 basic directions mentioned above are associated with the ancient Pa Kua or 8 Diagrams (trigrams) shown below, which represent the fundamental states of nature and their evolution. They are the basis upon which the 64 Hexagrams (situations of change) of the "I Ching" were evolved.

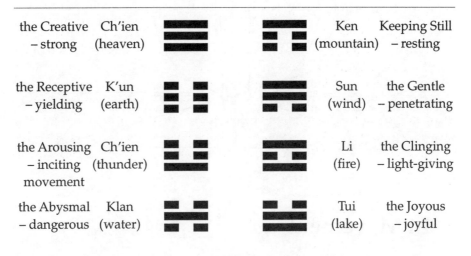

the Creative Ch'ien the Creative Ken Keeping Still
– strong (heaven) (mountain) – resting

the Receptive K'un Sun the Gentle
– yielding (earth) (wind) – penetrating

the Arousing Ch'ien Li the Clinging
– inciting (thunder) (fire) – light-giving
movement

the Abysmal Klan Tui the Joyous
– dangerous (water) (lake) – joyful

(For further details see "I Ching" Book 2, Wilhelm translation.)

Correspondingly there are said to be in T'ai-chi 8 basic types of movement, variously described as pushing, pulling, leaning, gathering, elbowing, spreading, expanding and grasping. Likewise there is a correspondence between the 5 basic positions and the 5 (Chinese) elements of nature and the compass points:

advance	– FIRE,	south	(summer)
retreat	– WATER,	north	(winter)
right side	– METAL,	west	(autumn)
left side	– WOOD,	east	(spring)
central equilibrium	– EARTH,	centre.	

Philosophically, Man himself stands at the centre, as he stands centrally and is the confluence of the influences of Heaven (Yang) and Earth (Yin): he is that 'ridgepole' – the link or mainstay, the creation. These are of course the most fundamental complementary opposites, both factually and symbolically. They create the Trinity which the Chinese called The Great Triad: Heaven, Earth,

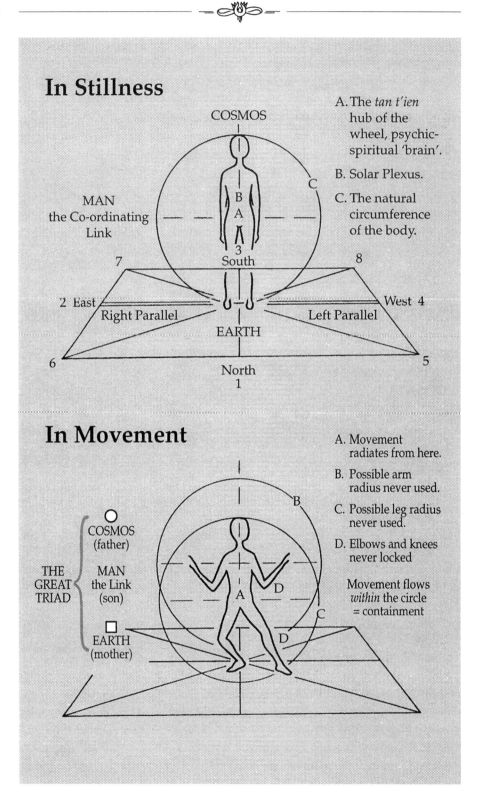

In Stillness

COSMOS

MAN
the Co-ordinating
Link

B
A
3
South

C

A. The *tan t'ien*
hub of the
wheel, psychic-
spiritual 'brain'.

B. Solar Plexus.

C. The natural
circumference
of the body.

7

8

2 East

Right Parallel

West 4

Left Parallel

EARTH

6

5

North
1

In Movement

COSMOS
(father)

THE
GREAT
TRIAD

MAN
the Link
(son)

EARTH
(mother)

B

A

D

C

D

A. Movement
radiates from here.

B. Possible arm
radius never used.

C. Possible leg radius
never used.

D. Elbows and knees
never locked

Movement flows
within the circle
= containment

and Man – the coordinating factor (the Son). In T'ai-chi Ch'uan and all arts, this Trinity can be understood as Spirit, Matter and Mind.

The construction of T'ai-chi Ch'uan aims to create perfect dynamic balance in Man's suspension between the opposite but complementary forces of Yin and Yang, vertically, horizontally and spacially, by the experience of coordinating the 8 basic movements and stepping through the 5 basic positions:

The 8 movements and the 5 directions, totalling 13, is significantly the total number of sequences to be mastered in the complete Yang Form (in this School). The first half of the cycle which I call Descent into Matter, comprises 5 sequences (2 in Part 1., 3 in Part 2). The spiritual number of Man is 5, i.e. 4 elements of the earthly personality + the self-directing mind/spirit consciousness, and indicated by the number of fingers or toes on each limb. It also represents the 5 elements of the Chinese system, the 5 limbs – head, arms and legs, and the 5 senses to be mastered. The second half of the cycle which I call Return to the Source comprises 8 sequences, 8 being the number of equilibrium – "as above, so below" (Hermes), of evolution, the movement of creative energy, the spirallic movement of cycles. The symbols of the second half and the conclusion of the cycle thus indicate the bringing about of balance and regeneration. There are other more obscure Chinese cultural perceptions of number 13 which are of less meaning for us. Numerology is of course always highly significant, and this aspect alone provides much illumination of the cosmic conception of the art.

As with the legs, the arms and hands express the alternations of Yin and Yang, yielding and firm, curving and pressing through space like swimming in air. Radiating from the spine and the *tan t'ien*, the 'hub of the wheel', movement flows to and out of the fingertips through the curved, spirallic development which is characteristic of T'ai-chi. Never over-extended or over-developed, the arms ride comfortably *within* their natural diameter-range, coming together and drawing apart, and reflecting in their soft yet powerful containment, projection and release the Taoist concept of strength in the understatement. Lao Tzu says "A man with insight knows that to keep under is to endure".[1]

Energy Currents

As implied earlier, of vital importance in this whole process is the area of confluence of the influences of Heaven (Yang) and Earth (Yin). This major area of interaction of energies in the body is called by the Chinese the *tan t'ien* or alchemists' 'field of the elixir', the Japanese *hara*. Broadly speaking, it is the area between the Solar Plexus and just below the navel, sometimes called the spiritual/psychic 'brain'.

---

[1] "The Way of Life According to Lao Tzu", ch.36, Brynner trans.

All body movement, initiated by the mind through the nervous system, originates physically in the nerve plexi of the spine and more specifically in the lumbar region associated with the Solar Plexus. Through this area, both within the body and in the auric field, energies are passed and redistributed according to need, not only the vitality of the etheric vibration (the support system of the physical body) but of mental directive including imagery, feeling and emotion, colour and sound vibrations. Although developed by Chinese Buddhists in recent centuries, much of this healing knowledge has since been lost, and needs to be recovered and revived in the mature schools of T'ai-chi Ch'uan for the particular benefit of the new Age. (The T'ai-chi as received by the Western world has been largely of martial perspective. Any self defence orientation is contrary to the essential nature of the art and will have to be filtered out, as it has no place in the Age of the Brotherhood of Man.)

The in and out flowing of energy incurred by the coordinated rhythms of body and breath, greatly heightens tactile sensitivity particularly in the hands owing to the use of the open palm (occasionally fisted). In the breathing discipline of The Healing School of T'ai-Chi (and the London School), all movements ride specifically on in or out breaths. In most schools today breathing is not so directed, the technique having been lost (not having been handed down), never acquired and mastered, or simply rejected. Without it there is too little power for the mind to ride comfortably upon or to generate either satisfactory rhythm or maximum healing benefit. (More on this in the next Chapter.)

Heightened sensitivity in the hands and throughout the body becomes possible only as one relaxes muscles and allows energy to flow freely through the joints, and ceases to force or pressure the activity in any way. It is facilitated by the body rooting and centring which enables 'emptying' of superfluous tension (i.e. over-contraction), and allows the body to be increasingly experienced as *less substantial*, while the atmosphere in which one 'swims' becomes *more* substantial: In heightened awareness, body and atmosphere are experienced as yet another pair of complementary opposites – an integral part of each other, interchangeable, and ultimately beyond delineation. In the natural world, this most intimate of all possible experiences is *the essence of unconditional love*.

This experiencing through the playing and manipulating of fine etheric energies is the key to and beginning of the real essence and charisma of T'ai-chi: It is possible to create, via the rhythmic ebb and flow of *all* the subtle/ spiritual vehicles through the centred 'location' of the body framework, riding on the breath, increasingly powerful currents of energy, and vortices which by virtue of subtle rhythm can attain a common centre of alignment, or centre of gravity. These movements are not merely within the more obvious lower subplanes of the etheric field (which include the meridians of *ch'i*) but involve the whole etheric, astral (emotional), mental and higher spiritual vehicles, the *chakras*, psychic body (the 8th vehicle) and the greater auric field. It is necess. to understand that the etheric energy field is actually the invisible aspect of th physical body (= solid, liquid and gas), and that it is comprised of basically 4 sub-planes: these are the 'etheric double' or cell-by-cell etheric framework on which the physical structure is built (not the other way around), then the finer, fluid meridians of *ch'i*, broader flowing energy currents as illustrated in the colour drawing (opposite page 54) and finer swirling, cloudlike currents. (See Colour Chart of the 7 Dimensions of Being.)

Energy movements include both clockwise and anticlockwise currents swirling above and below the body and through the Solar Plexus in segment-like streams, rather like an orange. In the highly developed, healthy person who is fully receptive and attuned to Cosmic (particularly intuitive) as well as Earthly energies, Cosmic energy pours down around the head and down the front of the body, and is drawn in through the body centre to the Solar Plexus. Here it consolidates into one major stream, and rises through the nerve plexi (*nadis*) and *chakras* along the line of the spine, gathering and drawing up into it and purifying the energies residing in the sacral and base *chakras* (*Kundalini*). The rising energy radiates out via the head centres, and the diffused golden radiance of spiritualized thought can be seen or felt as a halo (nimbus) around the head. The energy then swirls down the back and again into the Solar Plexus, radiating out laterally forward to left and right, circling the body, and meeting again as a broad stream at the back before descending beneath the feet, drawing in the Earth energies and rising. (Colour illustration opposite page 54.)

Here we have a small indication of the great beauty and harmony which is the potential of all mankind, if only we can be disciplined and uplifted into the unity and flow of the One Life. AUM! The energy flows illustrate clearly that we are not isolated beings. They are the very life and source of our Being, through which we are nourished and cleansed, and linked with all life.

Most importantly, the energy flow described above (one of many) stirs and helps vivify the 7 major *chakras* or vital force centres which are the links between the subtle bodies, draws into its movement the focussed energies of the astral and mental bodies, releasing them into the physical (dense 'bottom end') structure of Man. In this way are affected the 7 endocrine glands, the hormone-producing glands which are the externalization of the *chakras* and therefore affect all human functioning. These glands are the pituitary (master gland), pineal, thyroid, thymus, pancreas, gonads and adrenals.

The so-called spleen centre is not a *chakra* but the externalization of the psychic body, the seat of clairvoyant potential. This is an 'animal' human faculty distinct from the psyche, inadvertently confused by earlier modern seers with the sacral *chakra* (see diagram). The psychic body is the essential communications link between the personality and the higher planes, and quite differ-

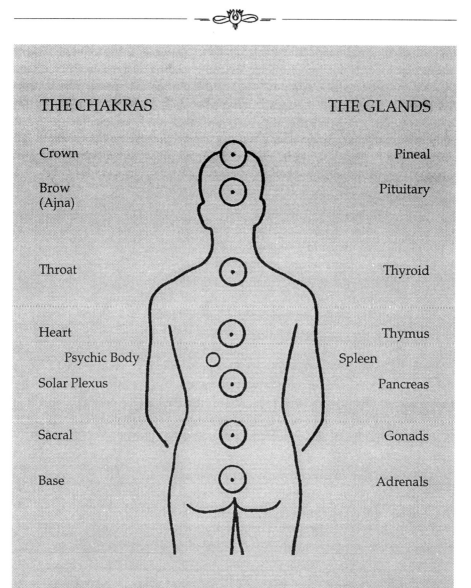

THE CHAKRAS   THE GLANDS

THE CHAKRAS	THE GLANDS
Crown	Pineal
Brow (Ajna)	Pituitary
Throat	Thyroid
Heart	Thymus
Psychic Body	Spleen
Solar Plexus	Pancreas
Sacral	Gonads
Base	Adrenals

THE SOLAR PLEXUS area is the spiritual/psychic 'brain' of Man, the confluence of Cosmic and Earthly forces, the blender and balancer of opposite influences, and the location of the physical and spiritual umbilical cord. Earth energy is drawn up via the feet, and Cosmic energy is drawn down via the head, meeting in the Solar Plexus area (*tan t'ien* or *hara*). In the spiritually developed person, Earth energies (*Kundalini*) are gathered, drawn up and purified through the higher vortices or *chakras*. This is 'the raising of *Kundalini*'. In the undeveloped person flows are small and poorly organized.

ent to the other 7 bodies. Initially a small egg-shaped body, it is stirred into pulsating activity and growth by the soul's upliftment through beauty and finer appreciation, gradually extending shimmering thread-like projections or tentacles from the highest etheric sub-plane into the astral body, the range depending upon individual capacity, and possibly (in rare cases) into the mental body. With this activity come the psychic faculties of clairvoyance, clairaudience, clairsentience, prophesy and healing, which, it should be stated, vary enormously in quality and range depending upon the spiritual unfoldment of each soul, and the development of the closely associated brow *chakra* ('third eye').

To return our thoughts to the energy flows, these are broad, full and uninterrupted in the highly developed person illustrated, where the body itself is stable and erect. The picture is very different in the average, certainly the undeveloped person. In being generally centred in consciousness in the personality and material interests, the body itself is then not so stable or erect, for the flows are constantly interrupted by the ego and external influences. Colours are darker, less vibrant or insignificant and feeble, with more reds and browns, less greens (= balance, harmony, growth, supply), and little of the higher Cosmic vibrations. The streams are smaller and lazier, more trailing. In being too concerned with the self and material interests, there is a lack of the expansion such as is shown in the colour plate. It is highly recommended that students acquaint themselves with the healing significance of colours – their physical, emotional and mental values and effects (see reading list).

Some knowledge of the energy streams, *chakras* and aura is essential to the full understanding of the nature and healing potency of T'ai-chi. We should not be limited to the hitherto available knowledge of acupuncture meridians, which although significant and valuable, is only a fraction of the situation, and stems from a particular cultural approach. The traditional view and teaching of *ch'i* is simple, clear yet limited in scope in my view, *ch'i* being regarded as an indefinable energy moving through certain Yin or Yang streams called meridians; the energy flow may be stimulated or sedated in any particular meridian either as the result of imbalance in the life, or through therapy to re-establish balance, i.e. the correct rhythm and pace of flow. This is the purpose of *ch'i-kung* training, whether for medical/health therapy, or self-defence 'power'.

We can in fact *create our own* meridians as we focus and move visualized energy streams, e.g. of light, as a meditation or self-healing process. Apart from acknowledging the external sources of *ch'i* in air (c. 80%, hence the importance of posture and breathing), food and water, the so-called 'development', focus and control of *ch'i* is generally confined within the area of the physical/etheric body framework in acupuncture, T'ai-chi and self-defence. The idea of 'developing *ch'i*' is considered an erroneous expression by myself; *ch'i* simply IS – we aim to *focus* it, and ensure that it maintains its appropriate rate of vibration or flow.

The human aura needs much more consideration in T'ai-chi. It is that area of electrical emanation which radiates (sometimes considerably in the advanced soul) *beyond* the dense body, and through which a person picks up or registers vibrations, both desirable and otherwise from around him – thoughts, feelings/ emotions, spiritual and psychic impressions. The etheric 'double' occupies the same space as the physical with an extra centimetre or two of radiation. The etheric field and the astral (emotional) and mental vehicles are much larger ovoid-shaped swirling energy fields full of colours and feeling/thought forms, being created and conditioned by the person's development.

It is essential for health that energy is allowed free passage *right through and out of the body,* so that all staleness is removed and constantly replenished with incoming life-force. In T'ai-chi this occurs especially through the hands and feet, the extremities, and greatly develops sensitivity and therefore healing ability. To merely direct energy around *inside* the body itself is to take in but fail or refuse to empty and ultimately *give out,* and leads to nervous tension and disease. It is an insular building-up 'against' life, instead of yielding and flow-ing with it. If one is to grow and develop, one must allow *space* in every part of one's being – *inner* space, otherwise there is no room for growth and inspira-tion, no room for that which is new and regenerative. *Energy flowing out initially carries the waste and the obsolete, but in due course of development emits the vibra-tions of good health and spirituality.* Containment of energy in the fisting of the hand in T'ai-chi is not a prohibiting of the flow, but a *creative focussing of energy* which must then be harmoniously directed and released according to the higher Will. This is an aspect which martially-oriented instructors need to address.

Colour, Imagery and Sound

The association between T'ai-chi form and subtle energy is very obvious to the seer (clairvoyant), and begs no less detailed study by modern clairvoyants than it did in past centuries. Inevitably with such studies, knowledge of the relation-ships between right thinking, right feeling, easy breathing and movement and *the corresponding vibrations of specific colours* will be brought forward, utilized and taught. Chinese Taoist and Buddhist seers knew of these things, as did the Egyptians and Greeks of past ages. Earlier in the present century much was recovered and projected by the spiritual teacher and seer Rudolf Steiner through his Eurythmy, and more research is now being undertaken into the value and use of sub-rays. (Eurythmy is a movement, colour and sound healing art and expression.)

Colour and imagery is an area of T'ai-chi of fundamental importance which needs much development. Together with music, colour is a major healing force for the emerging new Age, and we can see that as a composite fine art and therapy, T'ai-chi inevitably involves both. Study of the healing potential of col-ours and their visualization is of enormous therapeutic value, not only in basic self-healing, but in the development of the higher spiritual faculties.

All gestures, all movements of the body, produce qualities and degrees of refinements of colours in the body and aura in direct correspondence with the quality of feeling and thought behind them. Because of this fact, a clairvoyant who knows well the language of colour, and who *also* has a well developed *intuitive* faculty (spiritual) to correctly interpret their observations, can 'read' the whole nature, mood and development of a person. (See Part 2, Chapter 2 Research into the Auric Effects of T'ai-chi). It emphasizes the importance of unifying the whole activity of the personality in a positive and healthy way – the absorption, focus and release of the whole self in the matter of the moment, to nourish and heal by clearer and purer colour vibrations.

In T'ai-chi, the varying gestures of rising and falling, opening and closing, spiralling and circling can not only stimulate or sedate the existing energy streams, they can *purify the colour vibrations* of which they consist according to the degree of aspiration and heightened perception with which those gestures are expressed. The more perceptive we are, the more we will 'know' that a certain movement 'feels' a certain colour, and in due course of spiritual development we will even begin to 'see' it with etheric or astral (not physical) vision. It is an enrichment of our whole experience. We can feel for example, that horizontal movements or spreading the arms create green. This is because horizontal movements are actually a harmonizing of higher and lower energy vibrations – in terms of colour, the blending of blues and yellows. Green moves and enters the body horizontally, as can be seen in the colour plate, while the higher Cosmic vibrations of blue, indigo, violet, amethyst and magenta permeate from above, and the lower Earth vibrations of red, orange and yellow radiate from below.

This further emphasizes the importance of the Solar Plexus area as the great energy crucible of Man. From here, vibrations are distributed throughout the system through the activity of the *chakras,* and into the aura. We can also help ourselves on a practical level: on a cold day for example, or when feeling tired or depressed, red-orange rays may be visualized beneath and radiating upwards around the feet and body, and 'breathed in' via the feet to warm and revitalize the body: gently breathe in orange through the heels, drawing it up along the line of the breath within the back of the legs and body, allowing it to circle easily forward in the thorax, and breathing it out down the chest, abdomen and front of the legs and out of the soles of the feet. This is a refreshing, warming *ch'i-kung.*

Circulation may be stimulated and nourished by visualizing internal circulating energy streams of clear pink-red. The relaxing and cooling of body, emotion and thought may be assisted by the visualization of soft clear pastel blue-greens and associated natural images. These are useful and potentially powerful meditation exercises, for T'ai-chi students or anyone who cares to learn and apply the technique. This concentration is the directing of mental *ch'i*, a form of *ch'i-kung*.

Natural and flowing imagery is of a value not to be underestimated, for the use of thought and feeling can create either harmony and development, or disharmony and disease. This underlines the great importance of inspirational, creative and imaginative elements in the teaching of T'ai-chi forms; it is *not the form itself* which is ultimately important: good and beautiful form is the bi-product of *the quality of attunement* of thought and feeling.

Body movement needs to be consciously (but lightly and loosely) identified, i.e. felt, with the movements of life – grass waving with the breeze, clouds riding across the sky, the ebb and flow of the tides of the sea, the earth-mother nurturing and supporting her child, the cleansing purifying fire preparing the way for new life, the sowing of seeds in healthy soil, spreading the arms like the opening of the Way, opening the body to the warm rays of the Sun. In these images there is not only the natural release of the self; there is the essence of integration and upliftment of the soul. There is colour, rhythm and beauty.

Within the foreseeable future, music will come in, but not as an external melody or rhythm which would distract or dominate. This has unfortunately happened in Australia in some areas, reducing T'ai-chi to a merely pleasant workout, and preventing the higher development born of *listening and self-directing*. There is of course benefit in this, but the achievement remains on a superficial level. It would be less confusing, and more acceptable to me if such general practices were presented under another name – at least stated to be T'ai-chi *based*, or T'ai-chi *introductions*, and not T'ai-chi itself.

The music that will come in, and is indeed already in use, is of notes and harmonies and 'spaces' of a meditative nature which will lift the soul consciousness and permeate the subtle bodies with clearer, finer sounds and purer healing colours. In time, this will be more widely appreciated and evident. It must be nurtured with great care.

I am working with this. Music and sound must have clarity, simplicity, no melodies, and a spacial quality. The sustained flute sound is excellent, and violin, bells, gongs, and some synthesizer sounds may be suitable. Sounds can quietly and unobtrusively penetrate the aura, and flow *through* consciousness as a *subtle influence only*, the object being to facilitate greater release, particularly of mental activity, and enhance the whole experience. They must never be permitted to dominate the consciousness, as that is to relinquish the mental focus and directive. The human body is a musical instrument, the orchestra of the Soul, every cell and organ with its keynote, divinely ordained to transmit the flowing harmonies of the indwelling Spirit. When the whole human orchestra is in tune, and each instrument (cell, organ or part) is playing its part in harmony within the whole, we have true health.

Within moments of commencing the cycle, sometimes with the first gestures, the effect of sound upon movement may be evident. A distinct and often remarkable change occurs: face and body noticeably 'empty' as mental chatter subsides, and consciousness lifts and lightens into the intuitive, creative levels of flow. The smoothly penetrating vibrations of sound facilitate the lifting of the movements onto the etheric momentum.

Only advanced students with sufficient mastery of the Form can maintain the fine thread of directive awareness and not lose control. For this reason, the experience of sound is not offered until learning of the full cycle is completed – about two years. The meditative training of T'ai-chi being a process of *inner listening*, offering music too soon was proved to be a confusing distraction by leading the students too easily to surrender their wills to the music, or to create conflict in struggling to ignore it. The sustained focus and therefore power of the mind is a training in *focussing the will*, and is central to the whole practice of T'ai-chi. Experiences with sound are therefore *one aspect* of advanced training in this School as a development aid only, and always used with discrimination. Music and sound are a part of the ambient energies at the time of the practice – not rejected, not surrendered to, but *accepted as an integral part* of the experience. It must be remembered that T'ai-chi is itself music, and the art so created that advanced movers can perceive and *ride upon the inner sounds in the silence of their own creative activity*.

In summary, the overall task of T'ai-chi in the inner levels is to firmly establish, strengthen and purify all energy currents and rhythms, colour and sound qualities. This is the development of consciousness and personality, which influences the efficiency of all the circulatory systems of the physical body. It depends upon body rooting in balance with spiritual aspiration, moving through a light and free rhythmic carriage, and complete and natural permeation of fine mental directive and breathing – the key motivating factors.

In the course of development, the combination of all these factors has the extraordinary effect of allowing a shifting (transmuting) from the initial physical momentum of movement into an *etheric momentum*. This is an extension of what the Chinese called "directing the *ch'i*", but it is not a matter of 'doing' but of the 'being' which supersedes it as the personality (Tiger) is transmuted and transcended. It may be recognized as a subtle but distinct feeling of 'lifting off' and the movements apparently 'doing themselves', yet under the overall fine-line directive of the mind – the meditative awareness of the whole self.

Further Benefits

As a raising of the whole vibration of the personality, the etheric momentum is a very potent healing state. It is the product of long development via sensitive guidance and fine perception. It is the peak of T'ai-chi Ch'uan – the emptying of self to allow the attainment of T'ai-chi (integration, unity), perception of Tao (pure Being) and the emergence of what the Chinese called *tê*: intrinsic primor-

The Nature of Tê

Tê is usually translated as virtue or power, hence the translations of "Tao Tê Ching" as the Way of Virtue or the Way of Power. It does not refer to conventional virtue, for it has no moral overtones. It is an inner quality, potentiality or *latent power* existing in all creatures and things, and is a manifestation of Tao.

Being the inborn life-force, it can only be released and fully utilized if one returns to one's original nature. Once absolute quiet is achieved, this original nature shines through as a force. This is the purpose of T'ai-chi Ch'uan, to harmonize and integrate inner stillness with outer movement. Chuang Tzu says "Let your soul be wrapped in quiet, and your body will begin to take proper form" (Giles trans. Chap.11). Many subtle exercises and breathing techniques were designed to preserve the *tê*, especially sexual techniques, becoming very complex (and often very degenerate) over succeeding centuries.

Chuang Tzu defines *tê* or virtue as "the perfect attainment of harmony", and says that "there is nothing more fatal than intentional virtue". J.C.Cooper says of this:

> *It is sometimes suggested that the moral and ethical is ignored or neglected in Taoism, but this is a misunderstanding. There is no emphasis on morality because it is taken for granted; the stage of ethics is already surpassed. The Sage, the living example of the "Tê", is not a 'moral' man since morals do not enter his mind. He is already so perfectly adjusted and in such complete harmony with his surroundings that he acts with spontaneous perfection ... and all relative morality is adapted to the particular situation. ... Conscious virtue appears only in an already 'fallen' society and is symptomatic of spiritual malaise.*
> — "Taoism, the Way of the Mystic"

Taoism probably more than any other philosophy exposes and ridicules moral sham, and with characteristic light-heartedness and enthusiasm, for the Taoist Sage is by no means morbid and dull. He sees Man's moral sickness as rooted in *ignorance*, due to not understanding his true nature and identity with Tao. Hence Taoism has no doctrine of evil, original sin or vicarious redemption, and is free of the guilt complex which has bedevilled the Western mind. True Taoism has no doctrines at all, only principles.

"Taoism, The Mystical Way of Lao Tzu"
Beverley Milne

dial nature.[1] This state should not be confused with the more common state of rhythmic emotional euphoria, which is still 'doing' and still centred in indulging the personality ego (as in 'doing' T'ai-chi to recorded music).

The series of forms flows continuously like a free-flowing river, extending, withdrawing and revolving around and from a continuously travelling centre of alignment, the centre of gravity, and *within* the natural circumference or spacial range of the body. The characteristic vertical alignment of the spine, as in Yang style, is essential to all meditation; in rhythmic movement it makes possible deep relaxation, centring and poise essential for the flowing, fine balancing and permeating of energies at all levels. Like a living plant, each form grows out of that which has gone before, every aspect being at once both cause and effect. It is slow and peacefully 'beyond time', gentle but dynamic in its interplay, activating and reflecting the continuity of the Life Force, without beginning, without ending.

The characteristic slowness of T'ai-chi permits the full flavour to be appreciated, and the experience and energy value to be fully digested for maximum nourishment. Linked with this, its precision and linear simplicity are ideal for attaining detachment from the mental chatter of everyday affairs, and for focussing the mind to become aware of and to experience the quiet and subtle movements *within* – to exist in and to be aware of the *present moment*. Herbert Giles, translating and explaining the thoughts of the Taoist Sage Chuang Tzu, says

> When once inner repose has been established, outer movement
> results as a matter of necessity, without injury to the organism.

Moreover, as Chuang Tzu himself says, "to a mind that is still, the whole universe surrenders":

> The mind of the Sage being in repose becomes the
> mirror of the universe, the speculum of all creation.[2]

The forms should emerge as statements of awareness in time and space. They are often described as "moving stillness", for apart from helping to *engender* inner stillness, inner stillness is the pre-requisite for creative movement, a spiritual state of being which flows into and through physical form. All movement, all form, is therefore both movement and stillness, Yin and Yang, each being inherent in the other. In this way, grace and fluidity are brought to movement through the release of tension, extending awareness into all parts of the body and psyche through teaching the balancing of contained and distributed energy, of giving and receiving. Being unforced – effortless, the process of development is gradual and steady, and can lead (ideally) to the balanced energy which is complete integration of the Self.

---

[1] See "Taoism, The Mystical Way of Lao Tzu", p.10, and extracts on the opposite page.

[2] "Chuang Tzu", ch.13; he was the greatest disciple of Lao Tzu, 4th Century B.C.

The full benefits of T'ai-chi study and practice are too numerous to list here (if anywhere, but see Appendix A!) Although it is not a universal panacea, and every person is subject to particular limitations or personal maximum potential within the life (*karma*[1]), the potential of the art is not exaggerated – given good instruction, inspiration and sensitive response. General benefits notably include improved confidence, poise, emotional stability, mental clarity, better circulation and body tone, openness of joints and elasticity of muscles. Benefits naturally depend much upon quality of instruction. Currently instruction is often too limited in time and detail, as many instructors today are not really teachers, had inadequate training, have frequently never learnt a complete form (only a short form), and have little knowledge of meditation, posture or breathing.

Benefits to the soul life and fulfilment of creative potential however are of a different order to the general benefits, and beyond easy delineation. Nevertheless, in the posture and condition of the physical body we find the outward keys to general health in the complete individual, spiritually as well as physically: *As well as being the instrument of reception and experience of life, the body is,* and very often unwittingly, *the vehicle of outward expression of mental, emotional and soul responses, and the degree of perception of the spiritual life.*

Suggestions for further reading:

- ◆ Hara – the Vital Centre in Man – Karlfried von Durckheim (HarperCollins)
- ◆ Healing with Colour – Theo Gimbel (Simon & Schuster, Aust.)
- ◆ Know Yourself Through Colour – Marie Louise Lacy (Aquarian)
- ◆ The Science of Psychic Healing – Ramacharaka (Fowler Press)
- ◆ The Personal Aura – Dora van Gelder Kunz (Quest Books)
- ◆ Introduction to the Chakras – Peter Rendel (Aquarian)
- ◆ "I Ching" – translated by Richard Wilhelm (Penguin Arkana)
- ◆ Consulting the "I Ching" – Beverley Milne

---

[1] Karma – the law of return – we reap what we sow (root of reincarnation).

CHAPTER 4
Body Alignment and Breathing

Two most important factors in effective human functioning which do not receive nearly enough attention are good body alignment (posture) and breathing.

Good health is dependent upon several factors, including good posture, full body breathing, balanced nutrition, and balance in thought and feeling. All of these aspects are interdependent, but it is the physical body which is the framework in and through which everything operates. The body is a mirror reflection, the outer expression, whether we are aware of it or not, of all our ideas, attitudes and feelings. It presents to the world a picture of what we are and how we see ourselves. One who holds the body well is most likely also to have self-confidence and 'presence'.

The Vertical Spine

The vertically held spine allows the strengthening of muscles in the correct balance, especially important in the neck and lumbar spinal regions, and therefore maximum mobility and possibility of energy conservation and expression rather than tension and wastage. In the subtle anatomy it allows the major centres of vital force (*chakras*) maximum functional capacity – to absorb and distribute energy (*ch'i* or *prana*) from the subtler levels (spiritual resources, and derived from air, food and water) via the etheric 'double' into the physical body. Correspondingly it facilitates (along with energy movements) the necessary functioning of the 7 endocrine glands – which are the physical correspondence and expression of the major force centres. Poor posture blocks the free-flowing of these essential life forces.

Linked in importance with the vertical axis of the body are the two major horizontal axes, the shoulders and hips, linked and integrated by the fluid action of the waist centre. In normal activity, shoulders and hips should be kept level, for any tipping of the one will by correspondence automatically disturb the spine and affect the other.

Most alignment disturbance, caused initially by lack of awareness resulting in slouching, is physically due to habitually standing on one leg, or overworking one arm or one leg. When standing on one leg, apart from the effect upon the spine, the leg tends to rotate inwards and the buttocks outwards, causing the arch of the foot to weaken and collapse. Sloppy shoes and

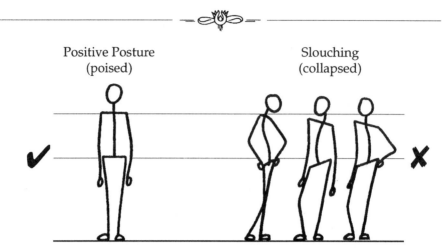

Positive Posture (poised)	Slouching (collapsed)
All in line and centrally balanced = equal contraction / relaxation ratio of muscle tension.	Weight dropped to one side, curvature of spine, neck and pelvic stress, loss of height, and fallen arches.

high heels also cause havoc all over the body. Since this is a very practical matter, here is a summary of

The Effects of Structural Collapse:

1. If the head falls forward, neck muscles are strained with the weight (c.5–7kgs.)

2. Back of neck nerve complex is constricted with hard muscle, therefore poor blood and oxygen supply to the head, leading to headache, migraine, blood pressure, dizziness, chronic fatigue, poor mental performance, affected eyes, ears and sinuses.

3. Neck angle constricts the throat, therefore poor breathing and voice production.

4. Causes spinal disturbance – hollowing of lumbar spine, weakening and therefore backache and spinal curvature.

5. Compressed chest causes shallow breathing, therefore poor oxygen supply and poor heart action.

6. Internal organs crushed downwards by the thoracic structure pressing inwards, therefore protruding abdomen.

7. Digestive track function inefficient, therefore constipation and 'wind'.

8. Reproductive organs affected; periods and childbirth difficult.

9. Legs affected: rotating inwards, knee damage, fallen arches, therefore weakened body support and more tensions.

The ideal is to stand relaxedly *between* the feet. Occasionally standing on one leg is harmless if the hips are level, the spine is well held, and you 'change legs'.

Good Standing Involves:

1. Weight equally between the feet,
2. Knee and hip joints open and mobile,
3. Pelvic area free of tension (especially abdomen and lumbar spine),
4. Feeling of upward lift (by a 'thread') through the head, neck and upper spine, keeping the body light and open,
5. Feeling of relaxation and downward movement (by a 'thread') through the base of the spine (coccyx).

In T'ai-chi exactly the same – spine upright, shoulders and hips level. The subtle feeling or idea of being drawn upwards through the crown of the head and downwards through the base of the spine, should open out the spine to its full length, removing any feeling of crumpledness.

Man however is designed to *move*, not to hold postures: Rather than stand unnecessarily, *sit down* (up straight!), maintaining a line of poise through the head and spine, with the buttocks well back in the chair, and keeping the thorax open and free.

Sitting Correctly

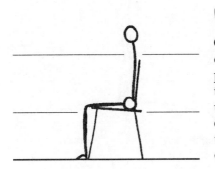

✔ **Positive Posture (poised)**

Centrally balanced. Spine rooted at the back of the chair, spine and head aligned and poised above. Chair is well designed so thighs are supported, and both feet flat upon the floor. Posture has centre and 'presence'. This is the correct meditation position – with palms down resting on thighs or resting upon each other.

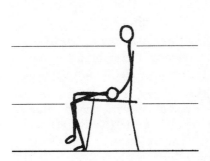

✘ **Slouching (collapsed)**

Neck crumpled, spine weakened, pressure of sacral (base) of the spine, strain in the back, shoulders and neck, rib cage crushing internal organs and impairing breathing, legs crossed = groin area closed and circulation inhibited, and leg weight trailing. No centre or presence.

Cosmic-Earthly Influences

Consider from the Cosmic viewpoint the position of Man as a physical being – a vertically designed and aligned creature. The feet are rooted to the Earth by the centrifugal force of gravity and the lower spine points downwards to the Earth centre and our physical origin. The head moves in space poised lightly over the upper or cervical spine, pointing upwards towards the heavens or outer Cosmos which is our spiritual origin and centre. With the feet – symbolically our Earth-nature, we are limited, earthbound; relatively, there is not far we can go. With the head – symbolically the Spirit-nature, we are unlimited, and with all creation before us to experience and through which to evolve.

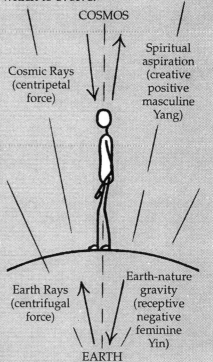

Consider the diagram of Man standing on the Earth:

a) In the sphere of Cosmic Energy movements, we are subject to the rays of light and wisdom pouring downwards from the outer Cosmos via the head centres, and to rays of centrifugal force radiating out from the Earth centre. Cosmic forces thus affect and enter the body from both above and below. Our very existence is the result of the interaction of these two forces.

b) In the sphere of personal awareness, we are spiritually aspiring or raising our thoughts, but also rooted by gravity into the Earth. Our interests therefore are movements in two basic directions: our aspirations, and finer more spiritual inclinations (Creative aspect) by which we attune ouselves and vibrate to a higher order of being, so facilitating our own evolving; our Earth nature, the physical nature (Receptive aspect) which is the essential counterpart of the spiritual Self which may, until we finds the balance, lead to indulgence in excesses, gross attitudes and behaviour.

All depends upon true understanding and balance in every avenue of life. Aspiration must be balanced with rootedness, and as this awareness develops, so can the Cosmic and Earth rays more effectively blend in one's being and positively stimulate growth.

"Body Alignment" (Positive Posture), Beverley Milne

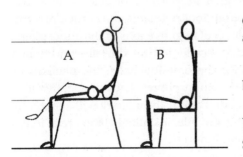

A   B

**✗ Slouch or discomfort
    inevitable**

Chairs badly designed to start with –
a) no 'space' for buttocks, seat flat and
   too long for the thighs, and no
   thigh support.
b) seat far too low, and no thigh support.

What can we do?

Sit on the edge, or find a real chair!

For a standing and sitting *ch'i-kung* exercise, see Appendix C, Exercise 4.

Good posture is also essential for effective full-body (abdominal-thoracic) breathing. This is impossible if the ribcage collapses into and crushes the chest cavity and internal organs. Unfortunately, many T'ai-chi instructors take far too seriously and without anatomical insight, an unfortunate (mistranslated or misinformed) directive of "The T'ai-chi Classics" (see page 59) that the chest should be sunk and the shoulders rounded. The object is supposedly to 'sink the *ch'i*', but in lacking subtlety of perception and conception, it all too often results in a slouching body, protruding abdomen, unfortunate lack of poise, and therefore *health liability*; if full breathing was practised this could hardly occur. There is often too much acceptance of gravity (rooting) in a collapsing way, and not enough suspension/polarity through the head. This lack of adequate suspension is indicative of lack of spiritual awareness and aspiration being expressed in terms of the physical. See box page opposite.

On the physical level, good breathing engenders deep relaxation and therefore the opening of the joints, allowing energy to travel freely and penetrate throughout the whole organism to cleanse, nourish and strengthen, and provide a subtle and rhythmic *internal massage*. Such natural internal massage helps prevent e.g. the formation of gall stones, which are structures caused by inhibited and therefore sluggish energy movement (inadequate flow); they should not occur if suitable exercise is taken, particularly if the body is well held, and full relaxed rhythmic breathing is practised, providing organ massage. Good breathing is vital for the effectiveness of the nourishment/elimination systems, keeping the blood pure and the body cells (especially the brain and nervous systems) well supplied with oxygen and other essential nutrients.

Most important of all, breathing is the major source (c.80%) of supply of vital force (*ch'i*) to the body, being inhaled with the breath, assimilated in the back of the neck at the top of the spine, stored in the Solar Plexus and distributed to every cell via the etheric counterpart of the nerves. The most abundant supply is of course in *fresh air*, notably in the mountains or near the sea, where we nowadays may say we have an abundance of *negative ions*. In the cities, where we are adversely affected by higher proportions of positive ions, our waterfalls, parks and gardens – even our indoor potplants, are particularly important in maintaining the necessary level of negative ions in the atmosphere. Abundance of positive ions are found especially in heated or air-conditioned buildings where the essential negative ions become attached to the metal ducts, artificial lighting, and dusty and smokey atmospheres. Lack of negative ions leads to fatigue, headaches and general depletion. Technology will eventually find a way of redressing the balance. Meanwhile, installing commercial ionizers could be considered for offices, restaurants etc.

Disease eventually emerges in the etheric/physical levels from inertia – lack of movement, blockage and misuse, hence the emphasis in T'ai-chi on relaxation and flow on mental/emotional as well as physical levels. Here again, true relaxation and flow cannot be attained where instructors proceed too quickly into the exercises and forms without careful and adequate preparation. This overrides the real needs of the students, creates stress in learning, and is generally self-indulgent for the instructor and poorly productive for the student. As in any art or practice, full responsibility and care are required of both teachers and students if there is to be real benefit and achievement.

Specific Breathing / Movement Alignment

In T'ai-chi Ch'uan, the entire body should be released to breathe as a living whole through the rhythmic etheric/physical breathing intimately coordinated with movement. The best means of achieving this is for all movements *to ride specifically* on the continuous, circular in and out-flowing of the breath. Pressing, advancing and sinking movements are expressed with the outbreath, while opening, withdrawing and rising movements are expressed with the inbreath. Form thus emerges through mind, feeling and breath directed by the will.

In many schools today, this full discipline has been lost. Specific breathing is not given, the flow of breath being left for the student to find for himself. There is certain value in this for a period in early training, but many instructors refer to and teach little of breathing except that it is natural and relaxed, thereby virtually opting out of its real study and use. Consequently, movement is likely to remain on the level of slow-motion 'doing', and fail to achieve the maximum opening of the joints, and any truly easy and relaxed rhythm and the benefits it brings. I am willing to work with any T'ai-chi teacher wishing to make adjustments to recover the integrated breathing-movement of their Form; it is a challenging task, but quite possible to achieve.

It is abundantly clear that there is a distinct advantage and indeed *far greater power* in specific breathing/movement alignment. This integrative discipline, in which breathing becomes, *is* an intimate, inseparable and natural aspect of form – indeed its very life, ensures full lung capacity usage and cleansing, and establishes full-body rhythmic breathing, a vital part of T'ai-chi's thera-peutic value. Where no breathing regulation is taught, the chest is often sunk and shoulders rounded – frequently following traditional Chinese teaching (surely misunderstood) about 'sinking the *ch'i*', often causing a general lack of mobility across the shoulders and upper chest. Little more than the upper chest is affected by the shallow inbreaths, so that much stale air and waste gases are retained instead of being cleared out and replenished. (A student of mine in London had been taught elsewhere to imagine oranges under the armpits; it took us 6 months to free the rigidity in the shoulders and upper body. This is a pointer to the fact that teaching itself, quite apart from T'ai-chi proficiency, is an art and requires intelligent awareness!)

'Easy' non-regulated breathing has an *initial* value in catering for students whose etheric bodies and therefore the physical, joints etc. are very blocked. However, specific breathing-movement alignment training caters for the fuller unfolding and development of *all* students: The breathing being of vital impor-tance and easy to unstable, 'free breathing' is allowed with early form training in my School essentially to stir the etheric body and loosen its energies. Inte-grated breathing taught with the form *later*, will then not impose but grow natu-rally out of the student's experience.

Students of The Healing School of T'ai-Chi in Melbourne are guided from commencement through a range of standing-on-the-spot relaxation/medita-tion *ch'i-kung* exercises to align body and breath – exercises with imagery, col-our, feeling, body and breath (see exercises in Appendix C). A wide and enjoy-able range of these is taught with care in the first term, preparing body, feeling, mind and soul for the study of the Form itself. This introductory term is of broad and general value, not only for those who intend to continue into the study of the Form of T'ai-chi, but for many with breathing, heart, stress, co-ordination and a variety of needs of effective natural therapy.

Specific breathing with the T'ai-chi forms is given formally after at least a year of training, at the end of Part 2 (half the cycle, c. 15 minutes of form). By that time, owing to the exercises of breathing practised since commencement, much of the breathing and rhythm has already been absorbed and assimilated inadvertently, particularly through relating to the teacher's rhythm, and the group energy. In this way there is no imposition, though the student must ap-ply discipline to learn and integrate the breathing so that it becomes second nature. In the second half of the cycle breathing is taught comfortably with the forms. Advanced practice of course requires the full use of the breathing sys-tem, physically and metaphysically, and is so quiet and intimate as to be almost imperceptible.

Speed of movement is another important factor. The complete Yang Form cycle as taught in this School, riding upon the breath, takes an average of about 27 minutes. Students who have newly completed the cycle usually take be-

Early Taoist Breathing Techniques

The first Taoists were Quietists (6th Cent. B.C.), aiming to still the activities of both body and mind in order to focus consciousness within. They sought pure consciousness, removed from the complications and emotional disturbances of ordinary life, desiring to cleanse and purify the heart to be a fit home for the Spirit. The heart was believed to be the centre of thought.

The earliest Quietist School had two main disciplines which remained basic to later Taoists:

The Art of Mind – freed the mind (or heart) from emotion and desire so that it could return to and express its original purity – pure *being*.

The Art of Nurturing *Ch'i* – concerned with awareness and cultivation within oneself of *ch'i* – the life-breath (*prana, ki*) which exists everywhere in nature.

It was said that "the strong of will are those whose *ch'i* pervades the whole body down to the very toes and fingertips." ("Kuan Tzu", trans. Arthur Waley).

These subtle arts were greatly developed by the Taoists to achieve the state of 'creative quietism'. Forms of self-hypnosis were practised – sitting with a blank mind, blotting out the senses and outward forms – to become absorbed in the all-pervading Tao. This usually involved some form of breath control. Breathing exercises were designed to make the *ch'i* circulate as extensively as possible throughout the body. Vitality was drawn from the Earth through the feet adding to the *ch'i* already present in the body, and to assist this early Taoists meditated in a kneeling position seated on the soles of their feet (they used mats, not chairs in early times). This *ch'i* force was really the gathering and focussing of subtle energy by the mind and imagination. The novice had first to exercise and develop awareness through the physical breathing before graduating to the directing of *ch'i* by the mind.

A poem on meditative breathing by Ch'u Yuan (3rd Century B.C.) is called "Wandering in the Distance":

> *Eat six kinds of air and drink pure dew in order to preserve the purity of the soul. Breathe in the essence of the air and breathe the foul air out. The Tao is minute and without content, and yet it is large and without limit. Do not confuse your soul – it will be spontaneous. Concentrate on the breath and Tao will remain with you in the middle of the night.*

(Trans. Chang Chung-yuan)

"Taoism, The Mystical Way of Lao Tzu"
Beverley Milne

tween 25 and 27 minutes, while more developed students (and those with a slower natural metabolism) may take 27 to 30 minutes. Those who do not learn or do not apply the breathing could do it much faster, or slow it down to 35 minutes. However, specific breathing-movement alignment is a disciplined activity which is not possible to slow beyond a certain pace, its easy and smooth regulation being intimately associated with *individual metabolism*. To be *too* slow is to be 'doing' instead of 'being', forcing the breath, and can cause stress through tension build-up, possibly oxygen-jag. In the mature student who has been well taught, breathing is so interwoven with form as to be inseparable – as intimately natural as everyday breathing, yet rounder and longer, for the entire body breathes as a living whole.

It should be mentioned here also, that the form style referred to here involves the *full shifting of weight* in the legs in every movement, not only when lifting off the floor, and not the 70% – 30% weight shifting as in the form styles of many other schools. This latter shorter movement stems more from self-defence training than therapy, and where the pelvis is often thrust forward. *Full weight shifting allows full opening of the hip joints*, most essentially in the 'empty' or Yin leg and side, and facilitates therefore *full-body breathing* – i.e. a fairly complete emptying and filling of weight and energy through the rhythm.

Philosophy of Breathing

Lastly, without specific breathing/movement alignment, the attainment of subtle co-ordination, release and ultimate etheric momentum discussed on page 23, may not be reached. It is in these moments that a true sense of union may be experienced. Through the Breath of Life, which is metaphysical as well as physical, microcosm breathes with Macrocosm as the barriers of diversity and separateness melt and filter away. That which is within becomes without, and that which is without becomes within – ceaselessly interchangeable and boundaryless. Inner and outer are experienced as complementary aspects of the One: "the core and the surface are essentially the same" (Lao Tzu, Ch.1.).

To the Chinese, the inbreath was passive (Yin) and represented the feminine principle, the opening out and lifting up of the self in order to receive, the drawing in of Light or Life Force. The outbreath was active (Yang), the positive muscular action of the organism and creative outpouring of the Life Force. Western physiology has tended to view this oppositely, reflecting an 'in-breathing' material culture more strongly polarized towards 'getting and possessing' than towards giving. Factually and symbolically however, the inbreath is the indrawing of light and energy (vital force) for replenishment and renewal – the receptive element, and the outbreath is **a.** initially the expelling of darkness, staleness and disease from the organism, and **b.** eventually the radiating outwards of health or wholeness, the creative fruits of spiritual growth.

The more effective the breathing and consequently the whole circulatory and functional capacity, the healthier the person has become. Thereupon, as indicated, he 'breathes out' or radiates health and not sickness, and is a healthy and positive vibration for all around him – not just mankind, but for all other kingdoms of nature as well. Chuang Tzu says (4th Century B.C.):

Concentrate on the goal of meditation.
Do not listen with your ear but with your mind;
Not with your mind but with your breath.
Let hearing stop with your ear,
Let the mind stop with its images.
Breathing means to empty oneself and wait for Tao
("Chuang Tzu" Ch. 4)

Spiritually, breathing is thus the eternal fertilization and mystic communion of Spirit and matter. It is basic in meditation and spiritual training, and a key to higher spiritual powers.

So breathing in T'ai-chi Ch'uan means much more than physical respiration and physical values. Metaphysically it is a mental force, an idea, thought form or mental directive which is travelling via the energy streams throughout the body *at will*. Following this principle of thought-force, streams of light-energy can be specifically channelled through the body for self-healing (also absent healing), and may be visualized as radiant or fluorescent-like streams of white light (which embodies all colour vibrations) or a colour selected for its particular healing value.

Such is the nature of the Universal Breath (*Ch'i* or *Prana*), the activating life essence pervading all Nature. Through the gradual balancing of all energies at all levels of one's being (to the Chinese, the balancing of Yin and Yang, of *ch'i* flows), one may become 'a fountain that never dries'.

This is the secret of endurance.

For a more detailed explanation of the history and principles of Taoist Meditative Breathing, see Appendix D.

Suggestions for further reading:

◆ The Body Reveals – Kurtz and Prestera (HarperCollins)
◆ The Science of the Breath – Ramacharaka (Fowler Press)
◆ The Secrets of Chinese Meditation – Lu K'uan Yu (Rider)

CHAPTER 5
Further Spiritual Values

While preparing a stable and healthy body, one moves naturally towards the attainment of the inner powers of harmony, adaptability and endurance. This involves spiritual awareness as well as subtle physical, mental and emotional benefits.

The outwardly soft and yielding nature of T'ai-chi, in balance with its firm inner spiritual core of awareness, is its great strength. "To yield with life solves the insoluble" says Lao Tzu, for "the way to do is to be."[1] This blending way of 'being' is the highly creative state of *wu wei* (non-action or non-interference with natural order), the harmonious and spontaneous way of action which Taoists called 'creative quietism'.[2] So as an art of non-interference with natural processes, T'ai-chi is a natural form of healing as a steady *holistic* progress towards greater well-being and inner growth, as well as of both preventive and curative medicine *at all levels according to the nature and needs of the individual*. Certainly such is its potential. It also recognizes that the unfolding of the true nature of man (*tê*) is always a slow but sure process.

To step through the forms of T'ai-chi Ch'uan in awareness is to walk the Path of Life – the living Tao, the Way unique to every soul, for all life is movement and adaption to the circumstances of the moment, and not in any sense a static state. Such is the teaching also of the "I Ching". So the practice of T'ai-chi Ch'uan, imbued with inspired thinking and feeling, can lead to heightened spiritual perception: As one develops within its framework and flow, not only the body but the *sub*conscious as well as the conscious mind may be relaxed and centred, allowing the spiritual inflow (downpouring) and heightened perception of meditation. The student's attitude of mind and approach to life – the whole understanding and use of the power of thought and imagery, are thus of paramount importance. Good teachers of the art will have attained a fine degree of inner balance and perception themselves, and so be prepared to guide their students with knowledge and inspiration.

The spiritual 'objects' may then be summarized as the outward calm and inward stillness of integration, of self-realization, of mastership – through discipline, simplicity, and the discovery of one's physical/spiritual centre related to all other life. This latter aspect is most important: All nature is One and inter-

---

[1] "The Way of Life According to Lao Tzu", ch's.43, 47, Bynner trans.

[2] See "Taoism, The Mystical Way of Lao Tzu".

related, and so harmony achieved within the self will be (must be) reflected in harmonious interaction with the greater Life. Its attainment in any person will be marked by an aura of peace and humility.

At this time in the modern world, the 1990's, as we move through the dynamic transitional stages of preparation towards the Age of Aquarius – the coming Brotherhood of Man, the beauty of T'ai-chi or any great art lies not just in the inner growth and soul expression of individuals, but through them the building of a new and better world.

CHAPTER 6
Symbolism

It is fundamental to appreciate that *all body movements and gestures are the outward expression of inner symbols, archetypes and spiritual movements*, as well as *the body language of the individual psyche.*

Symbolically very rich, T'ai-chi Ch'uan is essentially imbued with spiritual, mythological, cosmological and numerological significance. Some of this has already been discussed with regard to the use of the ○ and the □, the correspondences of directions and elements, and in the previous chapter.

In embodying cycles within cycles and sequent change without beginning or end, the art undoubtedly reflects the Cosmic and evolutionary processes of life down to the tiniest details. Its subtle inner mysteries take many years of practice and perception to be revealed. It clearly reflects the journey of life, the progress of the soul through incarnations, and of universal evolution in both structural and spiritual development. In terms of one lifetime, the flow of forms reflects the processes of birth, childhood, adolescence, maturity, old age and eventual release. This release (or transition) is inevitably rebirth into yet another cycle, for such is the spiral of life. We are clearly not perfect at the conclusion of one Earth-life, whether long or short.

As a matter of spiritual science, it should be realized that not only the release at the conclusion of *one* life, but the release from physical rebirth altogether does not mean that one's evolution is complete in any way other than that pertaining to the physical world of Earth, for "in God's house there are many mansions"(Jesus). Therefore, my own teaching extends and expands upon the root Chinese philosophy and symbolism. Before release from the cycles of rebirth, as has been indicated, one must attain and express one's own unique Individuality – returning the fruits of one's labours and realization back into the world. Upon release from the material planes, one is yet far from Mastership in the higher sense, and with many more initiations and 'worlds' to master ahead. It should also be considered that the Higher Self of every living being *exists within the Godhead* (Tao) *and has never left it*. Our task is to *realize* this.

A Spiritual Progression

As a spiritual progression, T'ai-chi symbolizes at commencement the moment of creation and birth. In Chinese terms this is the emergence from Tao ('descent' from the Source) into T'ai-chi (the One) as the polarized movements of Yin and Yang (Unity manifest as diversity) activated by *ch'i* (life force). Ulti-

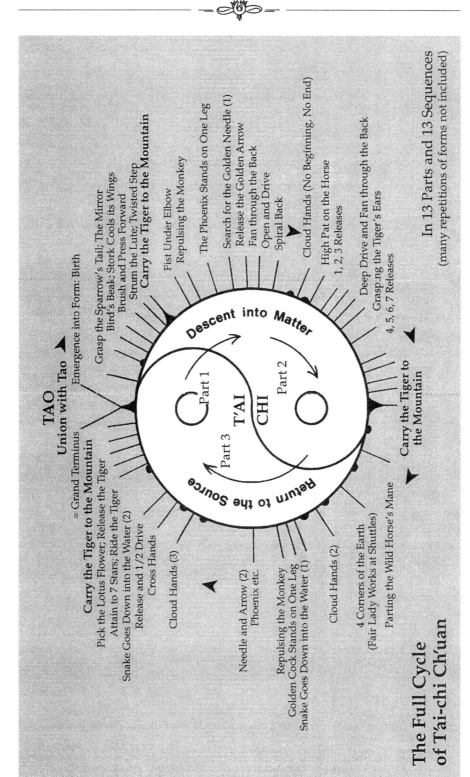

The Full Cycle
of T'ai-chi Ch'uan

TAO
Union with Tao
= Grand Terminus

Emergence into Form: Birth

Grasp the Sparrow's Tail; The Mirror
Bird's Beak; Stork Cools its Wings
Brush and Press Forward
Strum the Lute; Twisted Step
Carry the Tiger to the Mountain

Fist Under Elbow
Repulsing the Monkey

The Phoenix Stands on One Leg

Search for the Golden Needle (1)
Release the Golden Arrow
Fan through the Back
Open and Drive
Spiral Back

Cloud Hands (No Beginning, No End)

High Pat on the Horse
1, 2, 3 Releases

Deep Drive and Fan through the Back
Grasping the Tiger's Ears
4, 5, 6, 7 Releases

Carry the Tiger to the Mountain

Descent into Matter

Part 1

Part 2

T'AI
CHI

Part 3

Return to the Source

Carry the Tiger to the Mountain

Parting the Wild Horse's Mane

4 Corners of the Earth
(Fair Lady Works at Shuttles)

Cloud Hands (2)

Repulsing the Monkey
Golden Cock Stands on One Leg
Snake Goes Down into the Water (1)

Needle and Arrow (2)
Phoenix etc.

Cloud Hands (3)

Cross Hands
Release and 1/2 Drive
Snake Goes Down into the Water (2)
Attain to 7 Stars; Ride the Tiger
Pick the Lotus Flower; Release the Tiger
Carry the Tiger to the Mountain

In 13 Parts and 13 Sequences
(many repetitions of forms not included)

mately, 'reunion with Tao' is attained through the growth of awareness of the One Life and release from the cycles of rebirth into the physical world: this is the upward Spiritual Path and return to the Source. (See Cycle Chart opposite.)

This process of spiritual progression is presented in the story of "Monkey", a highly enjoyable and popular allegorical novel by Wu Ch'eng-en (translated into English by Arthur Waley). Monkey represents all of the weaknesses of human nature, the novel being the story of his corruption and ultimate redemption – the complete cycle of human evolution. We have a reference to this in the T'ai-chi form called Repulsing the Monkey, or the Monkey Steps.

The T'ai-chi art is a structured development like a play, being in fact a highly evolved creation mime play. It has three major phases or Parts, subdivided into 13 sequences or sub-phases – cycles within a cycle. Part 1 is the beginning, the introduction as in all art forms, the emergence of idea into form. All life is movement, and the opening form is conceived and born of the movement of mind and breath. The two short sequences comprising Part 1 establish the style and rhythmic dynamic of T'ai-chi's movement co-ordination.

Let us consider just a few aspects of the philosophy and symbolism of the opening movements. At the commencement of Part 1, the mover faces North (Heaven /Universal Law/the Creator/winter/night) symbolically in the stillness of the Tao. With the first inbreath, representing the opening of the whole personality (Yin) and receiving of the lifeforce (Yang), emerges the essence of T'ai-chi (the One) and the polarization of its forces (Yin and Yang) activated by the *ch'i*. This is the initial fertilization, followed by the first outbreath or creative outpouring – hence actual *movement* (lifting of the arms) should commence on the *outflowing* of the breath, as the body rides on the breath according to the mental directive. Each successive outbreath is a new creative expression.

At commencement, the body stands centred and at rest. Upon the first ourbreath the arms lift forward. On the following outbreath, both arms and legs polarize – weight shifting to one side and turning 90° to the right (one quarter), while one arm moves above and the other below to form a circle (Unity/Heaven): the dynamic interplay has begun. Turning to the right is to turn and face East, which also represents the Spring and dawn – regeneration and the beginning of a new cycle. Having turned one quarter, the mover flows on into facing the back diagonal or corner, and so on. In this way, the One (Unity at commencement) polarizes into two (Duality), which then divides into four – positing the 4 basic directions or sides of the square, and finally the diagonal – positing the total 8 directions. Hence we have the 4 sides and 4 corners upon which the stepping of the T'ai-chi is based. And so, together with the gradual circling and curving movement of the arms and body, movement from the Tao into multiplicity or "The 10,000 Things" is expressed. These are most beautiful and powerfully moving images with which to flow into the forms.

Then follows Grasping the Sparrow's Tail – an expansion of the body followed by closing and containment into a circle again, reflecting the 'newly born' attempt to adjust to the new experience of the complex world while still retaining consciousness of the Source (circle) and the desire to return to it. The palm of the hand then becomes The Mirror, a symbol of sincerity, and wisdom as in its qualities of immediacy and detachment it responds and reflects but retains nothing. Of particular importance is The Mirror's power to disperse evil, as it reflects the state and level of one's consciousness. Whether qualities of the personality or of the soul are perceived depends upon the degree of awareness of the viewer. This reminder gesture appears many times in the Form.

The Bird's Beak, called Single Whip in martial terminology owing to the cutting movement with the left hand, marks the end of the first phase or sequence. It concludes all ten sequences other than those which conclude the three Parts = Carry Tiger to the Mountain. Each sequence being unique in character according to its dynamics, purpose and context within the whole cycle, the Bird's Beak movement has subtle variations of meaning. The 5 fingertips of the right hand (pointing North/rest) all close together, symbolizing completing the statement of the sequence, and returning to stillness and rest in order to assimilate and integrate the experience. Chuang Tzu says:

> The bird opens its beak and sings its note,
> Then the beak comes together again in silence;
> So nature and the living meet together in stillness
> Like the closing of the bird's beak after its song.

This poem is also illustration to my own feeling of the T'ai-chi as a song cycle. Each 'song' has its own character and message, the threads of life (mind, breath and soul consciousness) flowing through them all. Like rivers and streams, large and small, drawn from and inevitably reuniting in the great ocean of life, each sequence represents a unique personality (lifetime) with its place and purpose in the series of experiences. Such views may yield much inspiration and understanding, especially when relating the flow of sequences to one's own experience of life.

Strum the Lute brings a musical image – release, relaxation and enjoyment of nature – to be without worldly desires. Most significant is the *inner* meaning of music, throughout the ages Man's divine aid in stirring the mind and inspiring the soul towards the Divine Source. Music is of divine origin, and is a means therefore of linking with the spirits or the gods; to the more developed Chinese it meant attunement with Natural Law: Tao. The movement itself involves a stepping back, a withdrawal following a forward, creative movement, thus indicating the essential rest, assimilation and consolidation complementary to all creative advance. (Modern name corruptions of Strum the Lute, rather lacking inner understanding, are Play the Fiddle or Strum Guitar.)

Turning then to the east (dawn/spring), the Stork (or Crane) Cools its Wings – a preparation before advancing. Brush and Press Forward represents advance and experience, always steady, modest and creative. The Twisted Step (side step) which follows is a preparation, a broadening of base to gather the energies and assess perspectives, the eye maintaining focus on the goal while awaiting the moment to move forward. The fisted right hand (focussed energy) is covered by the protective left hand. The left foot then stepping out provides the foundation for Open and Drive (martial term Parry and Punch), while the left hand clears the way and balances the fisted right hand as it drives forward. This symbolizes the importance of awaiting the right moment for action, of foundation, focus of energy, and clearing the way for effective expression of energy. The fist should *never* be seen or felt as negative or aggressive in any way, but totally creative, hence our use of root principle, non-martial terms.

Carry the Tiger to the Mountain concludes each of the three parts: Facing again to the North, the feminine element (Tiger/personality) acknowledges the masculine element (Spirit/creative), standing again upright and centred but feet apart, and the wrists crossed around the heart centre to 'close the circuits' while resting. As described earlier, the Tiger represents the incarnate self, the personality, which in travelling the earthly life must face and master all the elements and all situations, and is therefore subject to fatigue. While the Bird's Beak symbolizes rest for assimilation and attunement, this movement represents the end of a major phase. In terms of one lifetime, or spiritually the unfoldment of the soul, we might say that Part 1 represents childhood, Part 2 moves through the demands of adulthood to retirement from more 'worldly' activity, and Part 3 signifies the process of inner growth, completion and release from the Earth. Being earthly, the Tiger needs adequate rest, particularly at times of major transition, so the Spirit or soul 'carries' it to the Mountain for restoration of energies and re-alignment with the Tao. In miniature, we do this every night in sleep. The Chinese speak of the 5 Sacred Mountains as great storehouses of power, also symbolizing the heights of wisdom – being 'nearer' to Heaven, and far away from the distractions and impurities of city life. An excellent summary of this movement is in "I Ching" Hexagram 52, Keeping Still – The Mountain. In his commentary, translator Richard Wilhelm says

> *In its application to man, the hexagram turns upon the problem of achieving a quiet heart … True quiet means keeping still when the time has come to keep still, and going forward when the time has come to go forward. In this rest and movement are in agreement with the demands of the time, and thus there is light in life … Whoever acts from these deep levels makes no mistakes.*

Part 2 expresses through its three sequences the gradual and inevitable development into complexity – the further descent into Matter. It opens with repeated movements, an essential factor in the complete cycle, repetition being the very essence of life experience allowing strengthening, reinforcement and rest without the demands of new activity. They conclude in Fist Under Elbow, denoting energy containment before Repulsing the Monkey, or the Monkey Steps. These 5 gentle but firm backward-moving steps represent clarifying the mind and consciousness from disturbing elements, often called monkey thoughts by the Chinese, and refer to the personality's lack of self-discipline. As each hand press turns, the palm reveals the Mirror – mirroring the state of mind and soul. This is a powerful symbol, as it states that all our actions are actually and inherently reflecting our degree of awareness or lack of it. 5 is the occult number of Man: earth, water, fire, air + self-directing mind or free will, or the 4 limbs + the head. It also corresponds to the 5 Chinese elements, the 5 directions (see page 13) and the 5 senses, all of which energies and nature Man must come to appreciate and use creatively. 5 represents imperfection and testing, (= Earth + free will), and in requiring 5 steps states that such mastery is not achieved without patience and perseverance. The parallel foot stepping was the mark of the Confucian scholar.

Having prepared his state of mind and soul, Man is then represented by the yielding feminine symbol of the phoenix, which rises on one leg (Unity) facing and aspiring towards the North, Heaven and Universal Law. It is a symbol of gentleness, peerless beauty and happiness, was representative of the Empress and Heaven's favour and therefore a good omen for peace and prosperity. Most significantly, the phoenix symbolizes resurrection – death and rebirth by fire, and immortality. The Phoenix Standing on One Leg is an acknowledgement of Man's humble place in creation, rising open and receptive to the fertilizing and inspirational influences of the Creative Force. The image may thus have associations with early fertility rituals. (See colour frontispiece.)

Shortly afterwards there follows the Stork Cooling its Wings, a symbol of preparation for important creative activity; the stork is a wading bird, and so associated with water = wisdom. This leads into a highly symbolic and beautiful imagery in Looking for the Golden Needle at the Bottom of the Sea, or Searching for the Golden Needle.

Searching for the Golden Needle (the magic divining rod), and Releasing the Golden Arrow which is its development, are the outward movement reflections of inner symbols of the search into one's own divine well-springs of inner knowledge and being. It is the conscious and willing penetration into subconscious depths, encouraging the rising and emergence of submerged darkness to be faced and worked upon, and creative potential to be realized and directed. The tapping and raising of this inner knowledge, experience or perception into the light of conscious awareness is the springboard for its focussing (the hands lift and point to the brow centre, the eye of insight or 'third eye'), and its directed release as creative action. That which is golden is Yang – creative, positive.

The image of the needle gives much food for thought. It is a slender but strong penetrating instrument with the single eye of Unity and insight, the key and creative instrument of weaving the varied coloured threads of experience and attainment into the unique fabric of Individuality within the One Life. It symbolizes the eternal potential of fertilization of matter by Spirit – *potential* because the fruits of action depend for their quality upon inner calm, clarity and self-discipline. The movements therefore require full attention, directive, precision, patience and perseverance, the quiet preparedness to see the whole process through, with avoidance of presumption and care for detail and subtlety. Relating these movements to the "I Ching" Hexagram 48, 'Ching'– The Well is a deeply rewarding study. Water is a symbol of wisdom – simplicity, clarity, purity, nourishment (physical and spiritual), profundity, fluidity and adaptability – always finding its own level, seeking the lowest place, a cleanser and transformer, and potential of great power.

Cloud Hands (or waving your hands like clouds), sometimes called No Beginning, No End, follows this long sequence. Clouds are a transformational aspect of water (wisdom), and are a symbol of the ever-changing, elusive and mysterious Tao. This quiet sequence of side-stepping balances and blends the linear placing of the feet (Earth) with the circling motions of the hands (Heaven) through the *tan t'ien*, i.e. blending the circle and the square, or in more local terms – balancing the polarities through the Solar Plexus (personality centre) and the heart centre which is the home of the soul in Man. In following the revelations of the Needle and Arrow movements, Cloud Hands is a reminder that there is no beginning and no end in creation, for every moment is unique and every end is a beginning, every beginning an end. All achievements are relative, and must be correctly assimilated and carried forward through further effort and growth. This short but important sequence has a stabilizing influence, and prepares the way for the dynamic Release Sequence.

Part 2 culminates in the revolving, directing and energy-releasing dynamics of the Release (elsewhere misnomered 'kicking') Sequence. Commencing with High Pat on the Horse, we have a gentle but controlled approach to handling physical power (the horse; see Part 3 below). This lengthy series of forms reflects the peak of physical and generally outgoing requirements of adult life, and includes 7 strong and focussed releases of energy – standing and rooting on one leg, while the outflow of energy is directed through the raised leg and arms. They necessitate the most subtle body balancing and therefore emotional harmony, and quiet but strong breathing, steadily remaining within the immediate moment in consciousness. In riding upon the breath, this expression immediately and cumulatively reveals any tension and anxiety. It is of course the most difficult sequence to master, to attain and *sustain* inner and outer balance, and to weave into harmony within the fabric of the whole cycle.

Part 3, half of the complete cycle, has the remaining 8 sequences, and corresponds to the upward or return journey to the Source: it is the fuller awakening to the inner significance of Nature, and symbolizes the movement in consciousness towards and into the Spiritual Life. The short opening sequence repeats earlier movements, allowing a quiet breathing space before embarking upon new experiences.

Parting the Wild Horse's Mane is a subtle eastward-flowing parting or combing movement repeated 6 times, the 7th step facing again the Mirror. For each opening, combing movement forward there follows a quiet turning to the diagonal to hold the circle – containing and consolidating one's progress. Number 7 signifies spiritual power and the completion of a cycle (6 = harmony, love and beauty, + Spirit manifest), as we find in the colour spectrum, musical scale, *chakras* and endocrine glands, phases of the moon and other correspondences, 7 being the union of Spirit (3) and Matter (4). The horse is a symbol of inherently good but untamed physical power, requiring a yielding, accommodating approach in order to bridle and harness its energy. This sequence teaches the wisdom and power of yielding and gentleness (Yin, feminine) in overcoming and mastering an aggressive or intractable force (Yang, masculine), the 7 steps embodying patience, love and unswerving dedication.

The very contrasting sequence which follows features a flowing in and out between the pivotal centre and the diagonals: The Four Corners of the Earth symbolizes the balancing of energy expressed outwardly (pressing/giving and breathing out to the diagonal/world) with energy retained for one's own health and well-being (breathing out into the held circle of containment). Our earthly existence is already testimony to our having 'moved out' from the Source into creation, and the stepping outwards to the four corners symbolizes our earthly travelling outwards for experience and expression – literally, or in thought and feeling, followed by withdrawal to integrate those experiences. It is yet another expression of balancing activity with rest. Ultimately, the key is to remain in the centre in consciousness – the essence of meditation which teaches detachment and inner quiet. Lao Tzu says

> *Rather abide*
> *At the centre of your being;*
> *For the more you leave it, the less you learn …*
> *The way to do is to be.*

(Ch.47, Bynner Trans.)

This sequence is also called Jade Girl (or Fair Lady) Works at Shuttles, the jade girl being a serving maid to the gods, and the shuttles referring to the weaving in and out movement structure.

It is interesting to note in these last two sequences (Horse's Mane and Four Corners), that Holding the Circle occurs very frequently. This is a clear indication of Spirit consciousness and recognition of the importance of unifying the energies. Again, circling is characteristic of the Cloud Hands sequence which follows Four Corners: Although being in a later, more mature context within the process, we have the same reminder that all is relative, and progress made must be accepted with humility and assimilated. The clarity and attunement achieved in Cloud Hands thus prepares the way for one of the most important and colourful symbols in the T'ai-chi Form.

Having evolved through long trials and transitions, the moments of inner awakening often called 'second birth' or being 'reborn in the Spirit' are the rebirths into ever higher states of consciousness. Minor transformations occur throughout evolution, but a major one is an initiation, a shift onto a distinctly higher arc of being with all its adjustments and responsibilities. In T'ai-chi, the Snake Goes Down into the Water emerging transformed into the Golden Cock Standing on One Leg, represents such an initiation. Water being the symbol of wisdom, these movements represent in particular the purifying, baptising and transforming agency. The snake is a symbol of rebirth, able to shed that which is outworn and obsolete, of knowledge transmuted into wisdom.

Correspondingly, we can only attain to higher consciousness, or transmute knowledge into wisdom, to the degree that we are able to relinquish the hold of the material and transient – selfishness, arrogance, possessiveness – the Tiger's clinging to people, possessions, habits, beliefs and attitudes. In releasing the old, we create *space* for the emergence of new life and consciousness, symbolized in The Golden Cock Standing on One Leg. Both gold and cock are Yang, creative symbols. The cock notably heralds the dawn of a new day, but the day has yet to be lived; it is but another beginning.

Following this major transformation is a long series of repeated movements from the Monkey Steps, through the Phoenix, Needle and Arrow to Cloud Hands, as in Part 2. This repetition is a clear reminder that although the laws and conditions of life remain the same, *the context and import have changed*, for within time and space no repetition can ever be the same. The degree of spiritual awareness and therefore personal responsibilities are now much greater, and the fact is underlined that it is not the circumstance or situation which is most important, but *our response to it* which is the indicator of our degree of mastery. This long sequence is important for consolidation, but more particularly for *sustaining focus and awareness*. In 'emptying' and flowing along rhythmically on the breath for this lengthening period, irrelevant thoughts or fatigue may disturb the continuity, and the movement unconsciously move into 'automatic pilot' and become mechanical. Cloud Hands serves as a safety valve, and prepares for the final two sequences.

The penultimate sequence opens with High Pat on the Horse, a gentle but controlled approach. Moving into Cross Hands, the energy is carefully contained, and then finally discharged in one single Release movement: this may correspond to the ultimate spiritual requirement (before final release from the Earth) of giving back to the world the fruits of one's unique evolved Individuality for all that the soul has received on its long journey to self-mastery. This contribution may or may not be recognized by the world. Following the Release, the Twisted Step represents a restraining pause leading into a small but focussed Half Drive downwards (called Punch in martial terms) with the fist. The fist symbolizes containment and focussed power, and should always be used creatively; it is used here to curb any remaining vestige of the ego. This is most important, as spiritual pride can so easily overtake an advanced soul.

The last sequence opens directly into the movement of ultimate transformation – the Snake Goes Down into the Water, and as before, the left hand (snake) turns a full circle up, over and then down through the cleansing and transforming water. In releasing the last attachments and desires of the material world, the hand now fists and rises, joined by the fisted right hand forming a cross under the left wrist, the right foot pointing forward. This firm position represents full mastery of the Tiger to rise to the highest level of achievement – Attain the 7 Stars, attunement with the Cosmos. One is now fully awakened in Spirit consciousness, for the 7 Stars correspond to the 7 major *chakras* – now vivified and in balance.

The Stork Spreads its Wings again, and the cycle culminates in the masterly expression of Riding the Tiger, a unique full-circle 'riding' turn (spin) which indeed requires years to master. It flows into another circling and gathering of energies called Picking the Lotus Flower, where a clear but unexpected slap on the foot (root) symbolically stirs the *Kundalini* (life force) to rise rapidly through the body and emerge through the crown *chakra*. This is the moment of 'sudden enlightenment'. The lotus, rooted in the darkness and mud, rises through the water of life (wisdom) to flower in immaculate beauty and perfection in the light. In so embodying past, present and future – root, flower and seed, it is a favoured Buddhist image of completeness, enlightenment and Eternal Life.

The enlightened soul or spirit may then Release the Tiger, which means release from the 'wheel of rebirth' (a Buddhist expression) and from the physical world to return to (according to your philosophy) the Tao, or be reborn into yet another cycle of experience – a higher arc of the great Spiral of Life. Such attainment of perfection is a most beautiful and radiant expression of light, love and spiritual harmonies. The movement is similar to Releasing the Arrow, but with both hands fisted: the 'arrow' fist turns and opens upwards to release (in early Chinese terms) the spirit-soul (*hun*) to be reunited with the Tao, while the earthly-soul (*p'o*) returns to the earth from whence it came. The shell of the Tiger completes the cycle movement with old repeated gestures, and is carried back to the Mountain for the last time. Although there were those who perceived it, reincarnation was not an indigenous belief; it came to China with Buddhism (as rebirth) at the beginning of the Christian era.

As stated earlier, it is known in spiritual science that not only the release at the conclusion of *one* life, but the release from physical rebirth altogether does not mean that one's evolution is complete in any way other than that pertaining to the Earth. In The Healing School of T'ai-Chi, class teaching extends and expands Chinese philosophy and symbolism to include general spiritual science, karma, and references to reincarnation when relevant.

As we have seen, the colourful and descriptive names found in this art are the keys to the inner nature of the forms if one seeks and perceives its holistic character. Many of these have survived 2,000 years or more. Interpretations may vary, but this is an area of deep riches and growing importance in pointing to and reflecting the Way of Life, and it is hoped that what is briefly offered here will serve to inspire and germinate further thought and investigation.

The martial remnants in T'ai-chi terminology as inherited in the Yang Form discussed in this book, were fortunately few, and I replaced them in the first years of teaching. This in no way altered the form of those movements, but opened the way to clearer understanding of the root meanings:

> Parry and Punch became Open and Drive Forward,
>
> Deep Punch became Deep Drive,
>
> Kick became Release,
>
> Twisting the Tiger's Ears became Grasping the Tiger's Ears,
>
> Punch $1/2$ Way Down became Drive $1/2$ Way Down,
>
> and   Shoot the Tiger became Release the Tiger.

Self-defence terms are physically, generally negatively oriented and assume aggression to be counteracted. The constant use of such terms in teaching is not only uninspiring, uncreative and unnecessary, but is reinforcing negatives in the mind and consciousness – quite contrary to the whole creative purpose of T'ai-chi as it has evolved. Characteristic examples from another London instructor's form include: Intercept and Punch, Chop Opponent with Fist, Punch to Opponent's Groin, and Step Forward and Strike with Fist.

In reviewing the whole cycle of the T'ai-chi Form, we see that the three Parts themselves correspond to The Great Triad – Heaven (the father, Yang), Earth (the mother, Yin), and Man representing Creation (the son) as the coordinating link in being born of both polarities. Likewise they correspond to the Universal Trinity, the Creator, Destroyer and Preserver of Hindu culture, the essential aspects of the universal Whole, the essential dynamic components of the One Life: T'ai-chi.

The cycle of T'ai-chi Ch'uan, born of the Breath of Life, begins and ends in Stillness, the state of Tao, the Divine Source. The more one develops within the art, the more the stillness of Tao-nature extends and permeates the Form and the life, and it is this ever-growing spiritual endowment which is its real beauty.

'The Dance of the Spirit'

Of great value and inspiration is to perceive and interpret the cycle as a symphony, as a poem, play or song cycle, as the changing colours of the spectrum, a painting, sculpture or dance creation. It is all these things, and much could be written on any of these relationships. It is a statement of experience, life and order written in the music of time and space. Much of its real beauty and wisdom is elusive and indefinable – the nature of Tao itself, and yet experienced and expressible in terms of the vibrations and atmosphere of the soul and spirit, to which the body-personality, the crucible, yields to receive and pour forth.

The human body itself is the most intricately complex and beautiful instrument upon which we play. Each living cell is constantly emitting its own sound vibration according to the strength and quality of its life force, each organ having its own inner director, unique frequency and keynote. In the truly healthy person, enlightened consciousness coheres and directs this orchestra of the soul, ensuring that every cell and organ maintains its functional integrity and vibrates in natural harmony within the whole. This is the very hum of life. Our vibrational link with the Cosmos, the components of this great orchestra blend together and vibrate 'at one' with all life. Its voiceless music is the rhythm of one's own unique microcosmic nature, and as we refine our instrument and vivify and evolve the activity of the *chakras*, psychic body and auric field we strengthen our links and attune to the Macrocosmic Music of the Spheres, which really does exist. This understanding is symbolized in Part 3, as we have said, in Attaining the 7 Stars – the vivifying of all seven major *chakras* which are radiantly 'open' and linking on the inner spiritual levels with all life, our Solar System, and the Christ and Logos.

T'ai-chi Ch'uan certainly embodies the complete system of both personal and universal relationships as does the "I Ching". As a practical, living experience and externalization of the wisdom within the "I Ching", it teaches how to recognize the meaning and trend of the moment, and to be so attuned with life and circumstance as to be always in the right place at the right time – thus the *wu wei* or 'creative quietism' of intuitively (spontaneously) acting in accordance with the Tao. The physically refined balanced design of T'ai-chi reflects, as has been indicated, the phases and experiences of life, their contrasts of endeavour and withdrawal, and the comforting familiarity of repetition which is necessary for all consolidation and growth. In time, the spirit and poetry of the art speaks for itself through feeling and intuition, especially if the soul is stirred by inspired guidance. (This is provided that style and forms are as 'pure' as possible, i.e. well balanced as a physical and psychological *development*, and not the inventions of an uninspired enthusiast!)

The art form of T'ai-chi Ch'uan is thus a school of spiritual understanding as well as physical reform. Interpretations vary, relating to every level of awareness and perspective. One's responses to experiencing the forms and the level and nature of teaching are direct reflections of such levels of consciousness. T'ai-chi is simply a mirror of life and awareness. The order, harmony and beauty of form in the physical sense is simply the outward expression of its higher spiritual conception – the one born of the other, "as above, so below" (Hermes).

It should be recognized that T'ai-chi Ch'uan is of a very different order to Hatha Yoga. As a reflection of the Chinese genius to conceive of and express infinity in a nutshell, it is a masterly conception and embodiment of the *whole* process of human experience, not merely one branch of it – as is Hatha Yoga a branch of the greater discipline, and as a living fluid form is still evolving in the hands of the dedicated. The quiet, fluid movements, subtlety, roundness and 'emptiness' of T'ai-chi have had a valuable impact upon Hatha Yoga in the hands of enlightened Western world Yoga teachers.

There can be little doubt that T'ai-chi is more suited to the needs of Western culture, certainly for the great majority, than the posturing and holding involved in Hatha Yoga. In India was the need to pull-up, draw and hold together, but in our world – a very 'in-breathing', possessing material culture with a too-high gravity centre and accompanying stress, is *the need to yield and flow with the power of the feminine.* All life is movement, and through the creative flow of T'ai-chi we can indeed discover and experience 'the dance of the spirit'.

Aids to Attunement

While discussing symbolism in T'ai-chi, it may be of interest and benefit here to share some further perceptions of facing the North direction (given to me by the T'ai-chi 'Archetype' in the inner planes), and the power of the candle. The following section is adapted from my book "Consulting the 'I Ching'".

Facing North

For thousands of years, to face to the North has for the Chinese been a mark of respect and humility, for it symbolically represented facing Heaven, i.e. to face the Will of Heaven or Universal Law, and the ancestors. It therefore has the meaning of aiding intuneness with the natural order and processes of life. For these reasons we face North symbolically if not in fact, for commencement of the T'ai-chi Form, and also when consulting the "I Ching". There are however deeper explanations which may be of interest and value here.

Manifesting on the higher planes of creation and linking us with the God-head, great hierarchies of Beings channel to us its outpourings of spiritual energies. Indeed the hierarchical systems on our Earth are reflections of these higher orders (albeit so often falling far short of their intentions), for such is the reality of "as above, so below". Speaking in terms of general esoteric tradition rather than the Chinese, these great Beings, known as Lords, have various responsibilities within the hierarchical system, as good leaders do in our world.

Of particular interest to us here are the four Lords or lesser Hierophants, working under the leadership of higher Hierophants, who are associated with our Earth; they are the Lords of the North, the South, the West and the East. Other Hierophants have other planetary connections. These great Beings, whose work is to serve and replenish the Earth, each bring their influence to bear for certain periods in due succession, when each one is more closely linked with the Earth. It is the Lord of the West who is the link with the higher hierarchies – who has the more open way to the Godhead. The energies received by Him are passed on to the Lord of the North to work upon and prepare for the Earth, and thence in turn to the Lords of the South and East.

The process involved is that of a rhythmic receiving of energies from the Cosmic Spirit, and the pouring of these energies through the etheric Centre of the Earth, i.e. the Spirit of the Earth upon which the physical form of our planet is built. If witnessed within the vibrations of the inner planes, there can be seen a working outward from the Centre of the Earth subtle petal-like formations (geometrically speaking) by which the energies of the four Lords are linked into the Earth and with each other. The energies first received by the Lord of the West are radiated in rhythmic waves to the Lord of the North, who transmits it in its Earth-charged condition to the Lords of the South and East in turn. The energies are thus passed through into the Earth plane by all four Lords together in wave sequence, a rhythmic flowing up and out from the Centre and down, up and down again and so on in great sweeping waves.

Having looked at the background, we can now consider and understand the symbolic reason for facing to the North in commencing the cycle of T'ai-chi Ch'uan, or in consulting the "I Ching":

Each successive Age has need of a particular kind of energy, or conversely expressed – each new dispensation or outpouring of power from the Godhead has to have its modifications to meet the requirements of a particular Age. For this reason, not only do the four Lords direct the energies in rhythmic sequence, but they also take it in turns to provide the modifications and their own more specific guiding influence of a particular quality.

During the Age of Pisces up to the present century, the ruling Lord of the Earth has been the Lord of the North, having been the foremost ruler since the era of the coming of the great Avatar, Jesus called the Christ. Previous to that time, during the age of Lao Tzu, Confucius, Buddha and Pythagoras, the Lord of the West was the foremost influence. Hence each ruling Lord is foremost for the period of an Age – between 2,000 and 3,000 years. In the dawning Age of Aquarius the movement is towards the South, and the focus of influence has already moved midway in this direction.

It can be readily seen therefore, that the purpose of facing North when commencing T'ai-chi is an aid to attunement within the Age now drawing towards its close. Within the incoming Age of Aquarius, the same aid might be derived in due course, if one feels the need, in facing to the South. Similarly in consulting the "I Ching", facing to the North is deeply symbolic not only of respect for the higher energies of Creation, but because of that factor an aid to attunement. Hence within the Age of Aquarius, one might commence the T'ai-chi facing South. This is a thought for your reflections.

In creating what became called the T'ai-chi Ch'uan, the mystic Chang San-feng may have had an intuitive awareness of these powers, but it was others who later developed these concepts in China. It is understood by myself however that Chang San-feng, whose personality was long ago integrated within his Soul consciousness, is now a Master on the inner planes, and a great guiding light and power behind (amongst other things) the present practise and development of T'ai-chi in the hands of enlightened teachers. He is the inspirator behind the T'ai-chi Archetype, a great body of wisdom and energy composed of T'ai-chi experts and vast numbers of other interested souls in the inner planes, from which those who are receptive to the higher teaching may draw.

How important is it then, to face to the North when commencing T'ai-chi or using the "I Ching"? These aspects of spiritual science are here given for two reasons for the sake of both knowledge and inspiration, and in order that the principles may be used with awareness as aids to attunement. The answer to this question is therefore relative to the needs of the individual. Performing the T'ai-chi or using the "I Ching" are not a matter of outward form. They are inner processes: if one is aligned to the inner planes of consciousness through one's concentration, one is in tune. It is the *quality of concentration* which is brought to bear within the activity which is important. Facing North, candles etc. are not essentials but aids to concentration and harmony.

The great value of aids lies in times when there is need to steady the mind, when one feels emotionally disturbed and 'off-beam', when the personality, especially the heavy body itself, is out of gear and needs more adherence to all that will set it into coordinated alignment and harmony.

If one is calm and detached, the aids are not necessary, though they may be used anyway. To 'step above' is the goal. When we have built the Bridge of Light and can create and maintain our link with our higher consciousness, the art of T'ai-chi and the Book will serve not so much as disciplines, but as companions on the path of life for their great well-springs of wisdom and inner joy.

The Candle

From time immemorial, the flame and later the candle has been identified with the Light which is essential for all Life in our world. An agent of purification and renewal, it was regarded with awe as the embodiment of divinity and a symbol of sacrifice and resurrection.

But most of all our candle flame is both physically and spiritually a microcosmic sun, a spark of the Great White Light. As the human body is a microcosmic reflection of the greater Cosmic Body, so is the tiny flame a miniature embodiment of the Sun of our planetary system, an outward reflection of that inner light which is the spiritual well-spring for the personality – the microcosmic projection of the Higher Self or Inner Sun. This inner light is our living link with the Infinite. Forever with us, we have only to identify with it and allow its radiance and wisdom to permeate our being and shine unimpeded.

From ancient times this living link with the Infinite, the candle, has been used throughout the world in places of ritual and worship. For those who feel deeply on soul wavelengths, it inspires peace and devotion, lifting the soul towards the higher arcs of being bathed in the protective radiance of its aura.

This protective quality of candlelight has evolved throughout the ages. During the many periods of great religious persecutions, people have met together in secret, often in hidden and dark places (like the Catacombs in Rome during the persecution of early Christians), and they have looked to the simple candle as that light of love and wisdom which has ever been shed in people's hearts. Such focus on but one little flame has endowed its life with a spiritual soul, like a book or holy relic which is the centre of touch and concentration. Its spiritual energy has thus become highly significant, so that the ordinary candle, even if held unlit, can give a subtle feeling of support and upliftment to the perceptive holder. It has values little realized by many, especially in the dark days of the year, or the periods of inner experience called 'the dark nights of the soul', for light (enlightenment) dispels darkness.

When performing the T'ai-chi, consulting the "I Ching" or engaging in meditation therefore, the presence of a candle burning will be understood as an aid to attunement by aiding the raising of the vibrations. In summary it is:

1. the bringer of light into darkness, the Truth which dispels the darkness in the soul

2. a symbol of our divinity

3. a symbol of unity and livingness

4. a source of protection on the Way

5. a cleanser and purifier, burning up the psychic dross which is released as we purify and grow spiritually

6. a reminder that that which is received (inspiration, inner growth) depends upon that which is given up, even as the flame gives and lives spiritually by the giving up and dying of the material.

Your own contemplation of the candlelight and its aura is recommended for the many perceptions which may emerge within your consciousness.

The reflections which follow may serve as a guide.

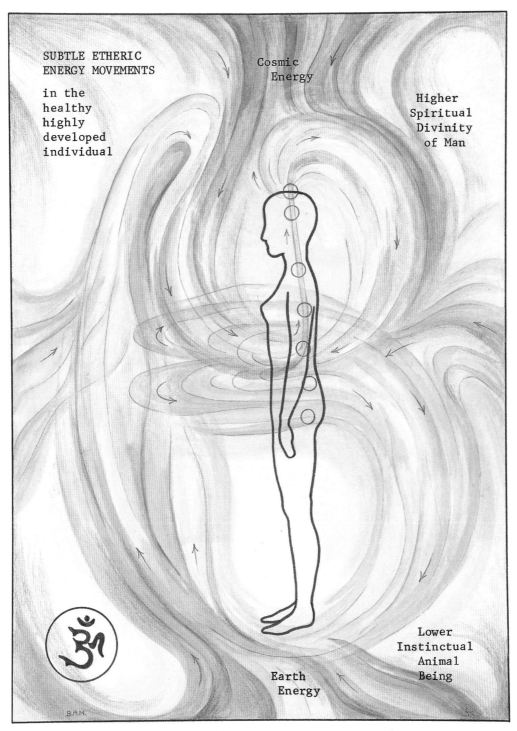

Illustration: Beverley Milne

Subtle Etheric Energy Movements

THE SEVEN DIMENSIONS OF BEING
and the Seven Bodies of Man

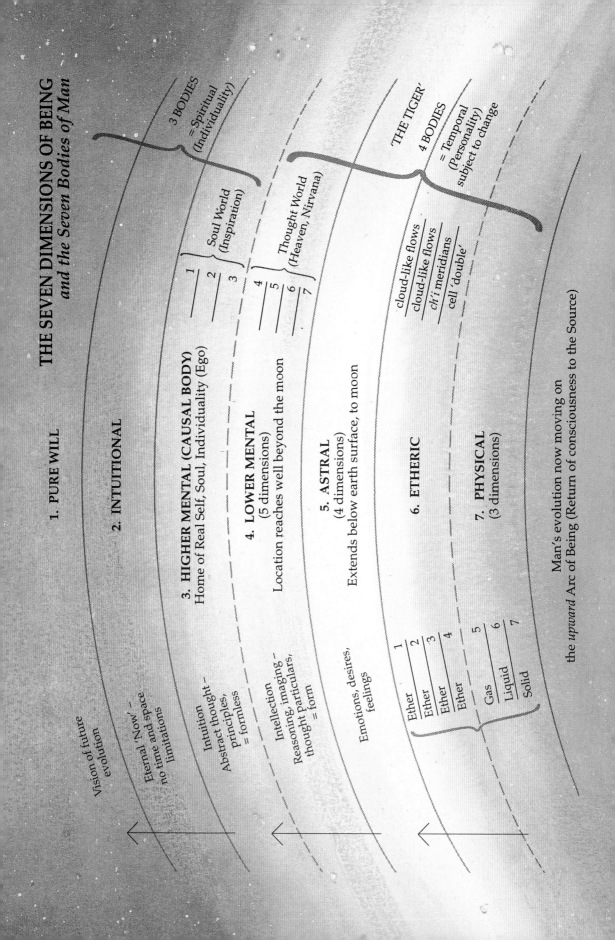

1. PURE WILL

Vision of future evolution

Eternal 'Now' – no time and space limitations

2. INTUITIONAL

Intuition – Abstract thought, principles, = formless

3. HIGHER MENTAL (CAUSAL BODY)
Home of Real Self, Soul, Individuality (Ego)

Intellection, imaging – Reasoning, particulars, thought = form

4. LOWER MENTAL
(5 dimensions)
Location reaches well beyond the moon

5. ASTRAL
(4 dimensions)
Extends below earth surface, to moon

Emotions, desires, feelings

6. ETHERIC

7. PHYSICAL
(3 dimensions)

3 BODIES
= Spiritual (Individuality)

Soul World (Inspiration)

1
2
3

Thought World (Heaven, Nirvana)

4
5
6
7

'THE TIGER'

4 BODIES
= Temporal (Personality) subject to change

cloud-like flows
cloud-like flows
ch'i meridians
cell 'double'

1 Ether
2 Ether
3 Ether
4 Ether
5 Gas
6 Liquid
7 Solid

Man's evolution now moving on the upward Arc of Being (Return of consciousness to the Source)

Notes

1. Divisions are of course very diagrammatic, and vary slightly with different schools of thought.

2. The Physical / Etheric is actually one dimension, the Physical.

3. The lower dimensions occupy largely the same space – not on top of one another, e.g. the Etheric extends throughout the Earth and beyond to form our atmosphere, and the Astral extends from below the Earth's surface to the vicinity of the Moon. Likewise in Man – solid, liquid and gas occupy the same space: we are not nearly as solid as we might think:

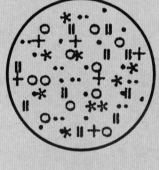

  .   physical matter

  o   etheric matter

  *   astral matter

  =   mental matter

  :   intuitive matter

  +   pure will matter

4. All dimensions are composed of 7 sub-spheres, which are as different in vibration as the solid, liquid and gas states which we know in this physical dimension, but which likewise blend into each other.

5. Lower Mental and Astral matter of Man (= thoughts and feelings) are very closely interpenetrating indeed.

6. All vibratory matter is *one whole*, and movements or disturbances in any particular vibration *affect* that whole, like the pebble falling into the pond creating waves.

7. Higher and Lower Mental matter in Man constitutes the Mind vehicle of Man and are basically one, but the Lower or intellective aspect is part of the Earth self, and the Higher or intuitive (Soul) is part of the Spirit Self. They are profoundly different in function, hence the division shown.

8. Little is known of the dimensions of Intuition and Pure Will.

Colour background by Helena Gibson

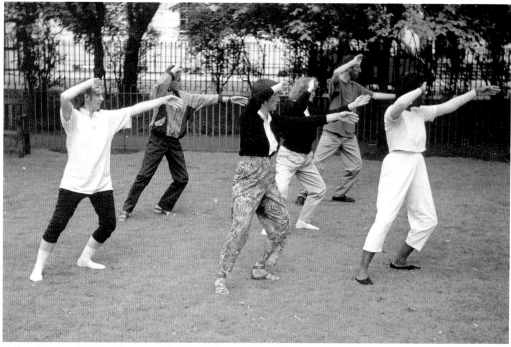

Releasing the Golden Arrow – Tavistock Square, London.

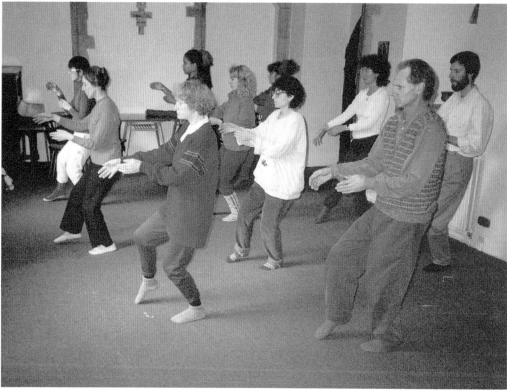

Weekend retreat practice at Allington Castle, Kent.

T'ai-chi Practice to the Right

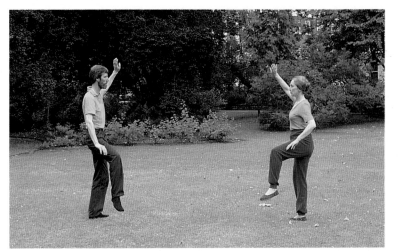

In these three photographs Peter is demonstrating the Left side form and Beverley the Right.

The Phoenix Stands on One Leg.

Photos: Ian Tapp

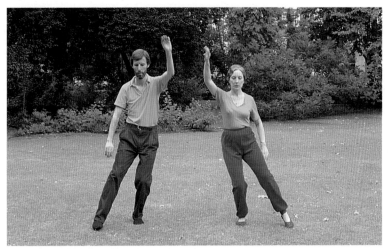

The Stork Cools its Wings.

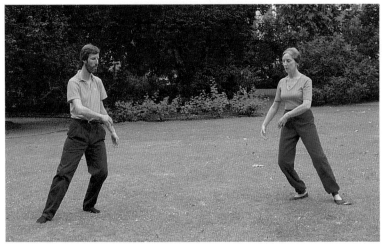

Gathering Energy.

Mirrors

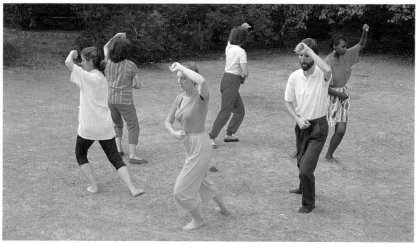

Grasping the Tiger's Ears.

Photos: Ian Tapp

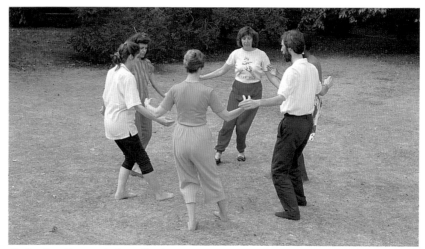

Gathering Energy before Closing, Part 2.

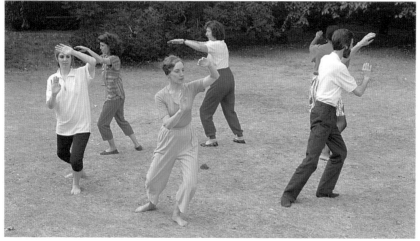

Four Corners of the Earth.

The Candle Dance

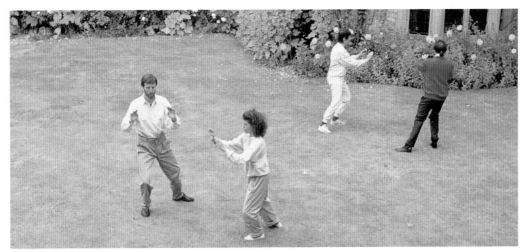

Pressing.

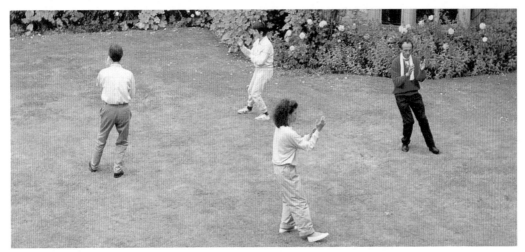

Strumming the Lute.

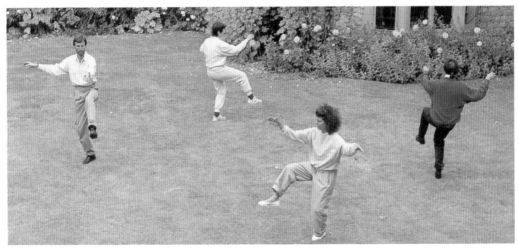

Releasing Energy.

Bi-Symmetry

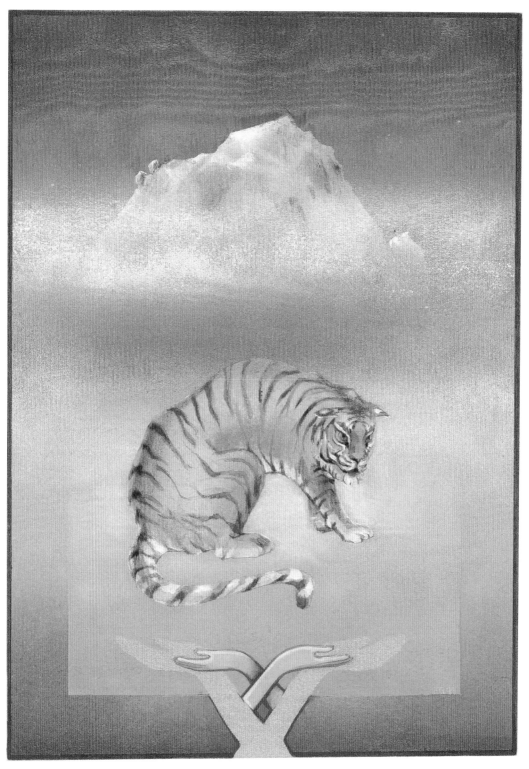

Silk screen / watercolour on moire silk paper by Helena Gibson.

Carry the Tiger to the Mountain

Thoughts for Meditation
THE CANDLE

So small, yet so brilliant and pure ...

In its simplicity and quietness,   not doing   but being,
    a model of naturalness,
        a symbol of unity –
           a single source and focus of light,
             a silent messenger –
                penetrating deep into the darkness
                bringing life, warmth and companionship ...

A unique integrity, bringing peace and comfort,
    the feeling of the warmth of the fireside ...

A living spiritual force,
    burning away the dross of the obsolete,
        discarded impurities of thought and feeling,
          cleansing,
            purifying our atmosphere,
              making softer, more wholesome,
            the aura and space beyond ...

Beaming out its protective auric arc,
    its golden rays of living light,
        pointing the Way ever upward to the heights ...

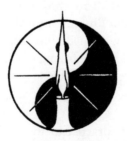

    A candle burns throughout all classes of The Healing School of T'ai-Chi, as it has always done during all meditation, spiritual teaching and other group sessions. In an art and healing work continually working with all the energies of concentration and meditation, relaxation and creative release, and of rhythm and harmony, it remains a centre of inspiration and a symbol of the true Way.

    For us, and all of those who are with us in spirit, our living flame is the symbol of the Inner Light, of Purification, Transmutation and Inner Peace.

May we all live, grow and be reborn
in the beauty of The Light

CHAPTER 7
Structure and Practice

Perspectives

The complete cycle of the long solo Form (108 forms) spans an average of 27 minutes to practice, depending upon the breathing, individual metabolism and form length of the cycle. It includes the originally designed repetitions which are reflections of nature and the phases of life, and therefore necessary for both physical and psychological balance. Studied first to 'the right' (one first turns to the right at commencement), the cycle should then be reversed in direction as in a mirror reflection and perfected to 'the left' (another 27 minutes) to experience and attain more complete balance. This allows not only muscular balance, but balance at all levels, especially in the more rounded use of both hemispheres of the brain.

A very interesting experiment was conducted by Maxwell Cade and Geoffrey Blundell with me in the later 1970's, using Mr Cade's newly designed Mind Mirror Electroencephalogram (E.E.G.), which could show clearly the brain rhythms of electrical activity originating in both hemispheres of the cortex. Seated comfortably in a chair beside the Mind Mirror with electrodes attached to my head, I moved into a meditative state, and mentally proceeded into 'the T'ai-chi experience'. The Mind Mirror showed the slowing of my brain rhythms from the normal waking Beta Rhythm into Alpha, then dropping into Theta Rhythm which is associated with meditation and creative inspiration. The machine displayed the gradual symmetrizing of the two hemispheres' activity. It was of course disappointing to be unable to see me for myself!

Quite often today, sadly, many instructors seem not to have even heard of practising T'ai-chi to 'the left'. Certain Chinese instructors and Western emulators have actually declined to practice to 'the left'. A recent Chinese acclaimed master in New York, although giving anatomical and other reasons, associated 'the left' practice with the Left-Hand Path, i.e. the path of evil or black magic, apparently failing to accept, face and work with the fact that the dark nature (earth ego) is an essential part of humanity and life. This is possibly due to the deep influence of Chinese religion and superstition. Mastership cannot be attained *without* embracing the darkness or fear within self and life, and transmuting it. To misunderstand this is to miss the whole underlying purpose of T'ai-chi and life itself. It is akin to suggesting that men should practice to 'the right' and women to 'the left' (– or vice versa?). One has only to recall that in all forms of movement and dance training, as obviously in piano playing, balanced expertise is required with both sides of the body.

When well integrated, the forms mastered to 'the right' and to 'the left' may then be practised 'in mirror' with a partner, where a new dimension is experienced by the requirement of yielding to the other person to form an external centre while maintaining one's own. This may require surrendering one's own form or correctness to accommodate the partner. Mirroring can thus be very challenging to the ego, for in the final analysis, one has only mastered the form *if one is able to give it up!* This ability indicates the mastery of the soul over the will of the personality. The practice of Mirrors is excellent training for all relationships, especially marriage! See colour plates.

There are also short forms of T'ai-chi which may take some 5, 10 or even 15 minutes to perform, but though now commonly available are not recommended for the serious student. It is a modern Western-world innovation (abbreviation) aimed at speedy results, originating in America, but widely popularized in China following Chairman Mao's directives for general exercise. In being chiefly a short-cut introduction and rhythmic physical/mental exercise (but good and valid as such) it lacks the repetitions, depth and balance of structure and design which is the essential nature of T'ai-chi Ch'uan, and therefore lacks finer therapeutic and spiritual value to quite a degree. Moreover, in studying a short form first, many sensitive students feel this lack of balance and do not continue, and thus barely meet the real art. It should be admitted however, that people get what they have earned, for we reap what we sow: those who do not seek at depth cannot receive at depth unless the teacher is at least offering it. A good student will usually find, sooner or later, a teacher who can fulfil his needs, and a good teacher draws those who can appreciate his offering.

It has been observed that in Australia, many people seem quite unaware that they are learning a short form (frequently the Beijing 24), and are often taught by people who have never even seen the complete cycle. It is in this area that 'doing' T'ai-chi to music has become common practice, a reason being given that Australians "will only come along and do it if they can do it to music". This is often true, for many are caught up in the superficial, but this will be discussed further in Chapter 8.

In style, that which is called the Yang, named after Yang Lu-chan the instructor who first introduced it publicly in Peking last century, is the most common and usually said to be the most 'authentic'. It had been handed down not from the monasteries, but via several generations of nobility who were interested in self-defence as well as health. Inevitably it now varies considerably in different schools, the art naturally having individualized in the various instructors of a number of generations according to ability and perception. The style of The Healing School of T'ai-Chi is Yang, stemming from Yang's grandson Yang Cheng-fu to Choy Hawk-peng (in Hong Kong) and his son Choy Kam-man. As indicated throughout this book, the work of this School embodies a revival of the essence and spirit of the inner teaching developed in the monasteries and temple schools, and is a vehicle for further holistic development. It is not the style which is the T'ai-chi, but the knowledge, insight and development which is brought to bear *through it.*

Less common styles were Wu (stemming from Yang), Ho and Sun. Yang, Wu, Peking, Wutan and Chen styles, and now Chairman Mao's National Style (short form) and Beijing (such as Beijing 24 short form) may be available today, and of varying therapeutic value.

It should be realized however that there are also now projected many self-styled or adapted-for-convenience styles and forms, even termed Yang, which do not adhere to its inherent characteristics of the vertical spine, subtlety, slowness and smooth continuity of movement. One of the problems is that since T'ai-chi has become more available and popularized, it has often been adopted and 'taught' by well-meaning but irresponsible teachers or students, including some yoga teachers, who have more enthusiasm than sense and humility, and who use T'ai-chi without proper training for a personal excursion in an 'in' subject; they are immature in both its knowledge and its practice. I have had experience of a number of such persons, who have thoughtlessly contributed to the degrading of the art. The lack of personal integrity shown (indeed selfishness) is very disappointing.

Another problem is that T'ai-chi has been and is projected in self-defence terms by instructors of self-defence arts, whose orientation, body-sensing and understanding, especially in the West, is far too masculine and physically based to appreciate T'ai-chi's intrinsic and yielding nature as a matter of *experience*, not merely intellection. True firmness or 'hardness', the bones and most basic Yang aspect of T'ai-chi, is the mastery of its *inner principles* – concerned with total harmony, not defensive fighting: it is the balance of 'inwardly firm, outwardly yielding' in accord with our essential nature. The appreciation that callisthenic therapeutic T'ai-chi is not a soft option but in fact a higher healing art, can only come with a higher perception of life. Therapeutic T'ai-chi and martial T'ai-chi (the latter actually intended as an application of the former's principles) have become as distinct and different as Taoist philosophy and later Taoist religion. Both of course are valid in their own way, but one might wish they had different names! In past times a student had to demonstrate a high standard of morals and ethics as well as fine technique before a responsible instructor would teach martial applications – a process of many years; they are dangerous in the hands of the unskilled. Few people learn effective (or otherwise) T'ai-chi self-defence applications nowadays anyway, and little but the terminology remains.

Happily for me, I have never been at all interested in self-defence except in the psychological aspect of learning and teaching the *outgrowing* of defensive and self-justificatory attitudes. In endeavouring to approach life as a master rather than a victim, I prefer to invest my energy in positive directions to find and maintain my own inner calm and detachment, and to creatively accept and work with life's circumstances as they come. This is of course the very essence of T'ai-chi.

Very valuable guidelines for the understanding and practice of T'ai-chi have been passed down through the centuries. These are "The T'ai-chi Classics", three treatises attributed to Wang Chung-yueh (14th Century). The essence and naturalness of the Tao, and the subtleties of movement, cause and effect, are succinctly expressed in short lines such as these:

> First in the will, then in the body.
>
> The breath moves the body, makes it pliable,
> so that it easily follows the will.
>
> In quietude as the mountain. In movement as a river.
>
> Standing as a poised scale. In action like a wheel.
>
> Strength issues from the back.
>
> First store, then issue.
>
> Through the curved seek the straight.
>
> Step as a cat walks. Use power as if drawing on silk.

The full study of T'ai-chi has obvious breadth of appeal, being at once physical, philosophical, creative, meditative and therapeutic. It brings relaxation to the body, release and upliftment to the emotions, peace to the mind, and inspiration to the soul through its inherent beauty and symbolism. A great advantage is that there is no age barrier. It is not an exertion but an unfolding, and therefore available to everyone including the elderly, and those with heart, breathing, circulatory, nervous and a great variety of other difficulties. It is especially valuable during pregnancy until close to term, and after birth. Few problems, such as severe arthritis in the knees, prohibit its practice.

The long structured discipline is not suitable for children. Children must be allowed to *be* children: they need full experiencing and enjoyment of their bodies and emotions in a full, broad and healthy way. Short exercises based upon the T'ai-chi principles can and should be available to them, their nature, colour and imagery suited to the age group. Most appropriate for children in The Healing School of T'ai-Chi is the *ch'i-kung* cycle of The 5 Animals Movements, of which details are given in Appendix B. Such classes for children are available in Melbourne, and are regarded as very important.

The time required to learn the basic structure of the cycle is of superficial importance, being relative to individual needs (not wants!) and perception, and to teaching methods. *Everything hinges upon finding the correct attitude of mind and acceptance of self (detachment), limitation and relaxation. It will* take at least 2 years to learn a complete long form.

Real attainment in the art, as in life, is a long process which cannot be hurried, and impossible through intellection and practice alone. T'ai-chi is not merely a physical/mental practice but the expression of a Way of Life, a Way of 'creative being' through the experiences of 'creative doing'. It is a Way through which we can enter within and express without in all levels of our being. An art of masterly subtlety, its profound wisdom and inner beauty can only be attained by full commitment to finding and walking that Way.

Spiritual Guidance through T'ai-chi

For the spiritually oriented student of T'ai-chi Ch'uan, the practice of the art itself can permit the reception of guidance from the Higher Self or other high energies. As an esoteric as much as an exoteric art, it is designed that this should occur. But it can occur *only* if the personality is sufficiently released and yielding to the higher Spirit. The vertical body alignment fundamental to all meditation practice, the opening of the joints allowing the energies free flow throughout the physical, the rooting of the body and lightness of the head and whole upper carriage, when set into subtle rhythmic flow, and *also completely and naturally aligned with and permeated by the breathing throughout,* has the extraordinary facility of allowing a shifting (transmuting) from the initial physical into an etherically-riding momentum. This etheric momentum is partly what the Chinese referred to as the directing of *ch'i,* though its real nature was commonly not (and still seems not) at all well understood. Some knowledge of subtle anatomy is essential to this understanding, along with meditation experience.

Lifting into the etheric momentum is a raising of the whole vibration of the vehicles of the personality, and therefore a very potent healing force in the causative sense. It may be recognized by a subtle but distinct feeling of 'lifting off', of the movements apparently 'doing themselves' yet under the overall direction of the mind and the awareness of the whole self. It is not a matter of 'doing' but of 'being', is the effect of release through very fine discipline, and is the key to the charisma of the art.

The rhythmic ebb and flow of all the vehicles through the 'location' of the physical body which is the framework base, riding on the ebb and flow of the breath, can create increasingly powerful currents of energy movements (*ch'i* or *prana*), and of vortices which can attain a common centre of alignment, or centre of gravity. This is the drawing into co-ordinated movement of the vehicles of the personality (physical, etheric, astral and mental) which are by their nature subject to the laws of change and therefore to malalignment. Obviously this rhythmic co-ordination greatly facilitates the development of the psychic body, spiritual faculties and *chakras* as *a natural unfoldment.* This is not a little the great healing value and *safety* of this highly evolved art – provided of course it is taught by one who understands its inner meaning.

To come to the kernel of this discussion: during the time of the full practice of T'ai-chi, guidance can be released from higher sources if one has made oneself receptive to them. If therefore, one has a problem regarding some matter or person, one should stand in meditation for a few moments as usual before commencing the cycle, contemplating this situation objectively, briefly but with focus. Then inwardly affirm "I commit this matter to my Soul and Higher Self for resolution". Finally, *completely release the question by breathing it in to the inner Self*, and proceed normally with the practice of the art. Do not expect the guidance to be forthcoming on the completion of the cycle. The Spirit will always take its own time in these things. Have faith, and leave the matter to be resolved within, knowing that when the time is right you will know intuitively what is necessary.

This is to realize the true potential of the art. The energy raised by oneself or by a group can also be directed, as determined before commencement, for absent healing – for a class colleague, friend or relative, or some group or nation. In the absence of a particular request, healing energy is *always* used by Spirit to good purpose. Many times the level of perceptive awareness will not be very high, or as high as one would wish, but one should try to avoid forming judgements, for they are not very constructive and can be limiting. In our world we are always subject to various forms of stress, personal and environmental, of feeling 'under the weather' or over-active often without any apparent reason, but the rhythmic discipline and swirling of the energies nevertheless bears much fruit in any case as preventive and curative medicine, improvement in general well-being to some degree, and in opening the personality gradually to inward realization and resolution of problems *in an unconscious way*. This process continues with the discipline of every practice.

In conclusion, it must be understood that this process is only really available to those who are not only striving for inner growth, but who have trained in the art sensitively (and with some inspiration) and acquired some real understanding of the nature of energy and the processes of relaxation and meditation. Few schools provide this. Indeed, there are few schools, for a great many instructors are part-time. Secondly, short forms of T'ai-chi are really basically healthy physical exercise (though by their nature far better than Western exercises like aerobics), and do not allow this degree of release of self and heightening of perception during practice.

The complete long form has the structure and length to allow full therapeutic value because it requires sustained, fine quality discipline, and thus makes possible this opening to the higher consciousness and fuller integration. But again this requires fine teaching, and full alignment with natural breathing throughout as a complete discipline. The keys are discipline, focus, release and rhythm, unified by the living breath.

CHAPTER 8
Teachers and Teaching

Seeking a Teacher

It will be clear that T'ai-chi cannot be learnt from a book. It is a living and very specific art. Students have individual abilities and problems, many of which they are unaware, and need inspiration and personal guidance in body alignment, relaxation and meditation, whatever the previous experience of these things. One also needs to perceive via personal example, and contact its inner Way of Life.

Being a highly complex and sensitive art (if communicated fully) instruction will vary as do the forms in different schools. The student should not accept any teacher, but make careful inquiries and possibly watch a class; then one may sense whether the energy, orientation and instruction are acceptable. However, good teachers draw students to them according to the degree of their own energy focus, and will be helpful and informative to inquirers.

Keys to a good teacher are:

◆ one who loves the art and the students, and therefore inspires respect as well as learning,

◆ who tries to *live* as well as give its philosophy,

◆ who has understanding and patience,

◆ who teaches clearly and thoroughly (not too fast), and is not doing 'his/her own thing' and expecting the students to follow as best they can,

◆ who is aware of good body alignment, relaxation, meditation and breathing processes, and communicates them,

◆ who has good knowledge of T'ai-chi's philosophy and its manifestations and living application in modern life (what the Chinese said or did is often irrelevant),

◆ who expresses his/her own reality and is not just a projection of their teacher (requires time and maturity),

◆ who does not dive into teaching forms at the first lesson (and if so, doesn't know what else to do).

Keys to a good school are:

◆ where classes are not crowded, but peaceful and well organized,

◆ where teacher and students get to *know* each other – each student being an individual, not just a body or face,

◆ where there is quiet, and sufficient room to move,

◆ where classes are conducted by qualified teachers (not students a few steps ahead),

◆ where there is a positive and creative atmosphere.

When you have found your teacher (and you may be led to the right one directly), place yourself fully and receptively into the teaching, but retain your own individuality and common sense. Remember that neither teacher nor student is perfect! You should sense intuitively if and when the time may come for you to move on.

The student's ability to learn depends upon the environment provided and the ability to *relate* to instruction, for learning proceeds from the known to the unknown. It may be said that a true teacher doesn't 'teach' anything, but has the *knowledge, technique, sensitivity and inspiration to inspire interest and therefore curiosity*, so that the student can identify with the teaching, feel the movements of realization and begin to apply them.

In the final analysis, much depends upon the student's own unfolding perception and application over months or years, even though the benefits should begin to be experienced from the very first lesson.

It is hardly possible however, for the full benefits of T'ai-chi to be expected via instructors who are inadequately trained or poor communicators (especially self-appointed enthusiasts). Too many communicators today are viewing, adopting and projecting the art from a personally undeveloped physical perspective, and are sometimes no more than 'bandwaggoners'. Some have simply shirked the discipline of essential training. Others quite honestly desire to share (and intention *is* important) but are nevertheless 'jumping the gun': too often they are the product of their instructor's failure to take responsibility to train them properly, or redirect them to another teacher who *will* (negligence or pride), or to recognize and tell them bluntly that they are not suited to it. Some are simply motivated by the desire to project *themselves*. T'ai-chi in this area is little more than doing the steps. Such is 'the way of the world', particularly the Western world – still largely asleep to the profound difference between 'doing' and 'being', and the importance of, as Lao Tzu says "to earn, not appropriate".

It is observed that in Australia (far more than in Britain) many teachers of T'ai-chi have learnt only shortened versions, some not even knowing of the existence of the complete form, or left side practice. There seems to be little knowledge of breathing or meditation, and little if any knowledge of the back-

To Teach or Not to Teach?
Shadow-band Energies: A Warning

A student desirous of teaching T'ai-chi proved to be quite unsuitable (for some years at least) although this was not accepted, having sought to impress and ingratiate by deception, and desiring to project herself as a centre of focus rather than the art as a service.

'Shadow-band' energies, which are negative, earth-bound and mischievous spirits including false 'guides', were hovering around this woman, impinging upon the aura and influencing her mind and emotions in a grey manner. Such energies are attracted to and feed upon the ego-centredness and physical-emotional propensities. In such instances, the true spiritual Guide and helpers are held at bay because of the person's use of *free will* to listen to the wrong voices.

Being unable at that time to recognize and face the reality of the ego's dominance and artificiality, there was an inability to accept the requirements and discipline of study. Following a period of difficulty and confrontation, this woman was obliged to leave the School, moving then to an 'easier', less discriminating and more impressionable climate of more physical orientation – a less aware and less demanding teacher who would (and did) admire, and was herself susceptible to admiration.

All students of the true Way of T'ai-chi must remain aware of its higher purpose – the integration and transmutation of the self. Moreover, one who would serve and teach others must first serve and teach himself, and continue to do so. As Lao Tzu said "one who knows his lot to be the lot of all other men is a safe man to guide them" (Ch. 13 Bynner trans.). The true way in all things is through self-honesty and discipline, even though one makes mistakes. In this way one earns and attracts spiritual protection through sincere endeavour and centredness, and 'shadow-band' energies will either not be attracted or not gain influence. Self-indulgence in any way opens the door to negative influences. We live in a world of cause and effect, and we reap what we ourselves sow.

This person achieved little in teaching, having attracted the easily impressed who fawn upon their leader, but will in time awaken to her folly, obliged to face the Self. We should remember that energies of thought and feeling, of good or ill, are instantly *multiplied* in the inner planes without our conscious knowledge. We have great power within our reach, to use for health and growth, or otherwise …

ground or philosophy of the art. Few seem able to explain correctly the meaning of T'ai-chi, and one lady, claiming to teach Yang style, inquired where one could learn Yin style! There is a great need in this country for not only *deeper, longer and more detailed study*, but for *taking greater responsibility in the art of teaching*, personal integrity, poise and reserve.

More fully and holistically trained teachers are needed and will emerge, who will require a high standard of expression in student attitudes as well as form movement technique. Technique without soul is not an art form. Teaching is also a profession which should always have and deserve a high standing, and as T'ai-chi is an evolved form of natural medicine relative to all people, training should be favourably comparable at all times with other schools of healing such as acupuncture (*not* the post graduate medical short courses!), osteopathy, chiropractic, naturopathy, homeopathy etc.

These statements are however intended more *to awaken and improve discrimination*, approaching the matter more from the grass roots, than to correct the superficial, for the superficial – in lacking the roots for growth, will ultimately die. It is for the student to raise his aspirations and expectancy, requiring a higher standard of teaching. Personally, I have always respected the perspectives and reality of other communicators, whatever the degree of awareness and wisdom, for every one of us is in the world to learn and to give. However, holding in mind the need *to earn, not appropriate*, I trust that my thoughts and my plea may help to awaken some instructors out of their complacency to develop their competence, and enrich what are too often otherwise empty forms. The importance of physical health is obvious to most people, but psychological balance and health, and most necessary creative (soul) expression are underestimated and underplayed in our culture.

As a weekly workout to music, currently available short versions of T'ai-chi with their rhythm and easy flow are certainly vastly better than Western exercising like aerobics (which is mechanical, overstimulating and generally blunting sensitivity), and as such they have much value. As a watered-down corruption of a truly beautiful art however, and a personality expression not attending to the higher needs of the soul, it is in my view not worthy of the name of T'ai-chi, though outwardly T'ai-chi in style. By its very name, T'ai-chi must embrace *the whole self*, even in a short form.

In some areas instructors are distinguished from their teacher, the former being part-time vehicles for passing on mainly physical forms, while under the direction of a (usually Chinese) teacher or master who is often abroad or interstate. This system may be genuine and well-organized, or may not. The fact is clear however that many students are receiving tuition (or copying) from well-meaning, maybe quite dedicated instructors who are in my view usually more the equivalent of the Chinese country 'bare-foot doctors' than properly qualified practitioners. Quality is sacrificed for quantity. Is this right, and is it necessary?

In any other form of natural medicine or therapy in our culture, complex practices, would we accept this? I suspect that this occurs because however beneficial, T'ai-chi is undertaken *as an option, not as an emergency.* Yet in other complex therapies or fine arts, years of detailed study both theory and practical are required. Indeed this was so in China, where T'ai-chi has long been a University faculty. In a more superficial culture, the physical 'body' of T'ai-chi seems easy prey for mere copiers.

Sadly, the above system seems to regard a student more as a body to be mobilized than an intelligent and sensitive personality to be appreciated and developed. Classes may be surprisingly inexpensive to attend, but one may pay the price in other ways. More people may be introduced to 'T'ai-chi' this way, but many may be disillusioned and not meet the real art. It is a good way to erode the standards of an art which took hundreds of years (modestly speaking) of careful nurturing to evolve. Some people today may object to the centuries of exclusive possession of T'ai-chi practice by the monasteries and Chinese élite, yet were it not so we would not have the art. This century's fragmentation of T'ai-chi by focussing disproportionately upon its physical form is symptomatic of modern materialism, and is contrary to the essence of T'ai-chi which speaks of *inner stillness* and 'falling back upon the root' – the *cause levels* of disease. It is akin to attending to the wound, the symptom, *without addressing the cause.*

One should also be wary of those who accept large numbers of students with the attitude that in due course many will drop out "and then I get down to the 'nitty gritty'". Interest in the needs of the individual should commence with the first contact, and no more students be accepted than shall be given proper care. Swami Vishnudevananda says

> *One can become a teacher very easily. To become a student takes a whole lifetime. The easiest thing in this world is to teach something one doesn't know and practice. The most difficult of all things is to practice what one preaches.*[1]

Teachers of T'ai-chi should in my view be *either* of full and detailed traditional training and its concepts and methods, and able to adapt it to our own cultural needs, *or* of full and detailed holistic training in the art as an instrument of healing. Other teachers may by training and experience be associated and work with both these approaches according to their contacts and individuality, and form a valuable bridge of conception and instruction. As we move forward into the New Age however, there will undoubtedly be, must be, more of the healers and a filtering out of the traditionalists. In any event, both knowledge and inspiration are essential if teachers (and therefore students) are to be in tune with the energies and needs of the times.

---

[1] "The Complete Illustrated Book of Yoga", p.254 (Julian Press Inc. N.Y.)

Never press an unprepared person into teaching you – one who has learnt the forms, but maybe not very well (you wouldn't know). That which 'looks good' is often wrong. Apart from knowledge and training, which includes much self-directed study and should in my view be not less than four years to allow for some maturity, there is that essential factor of *communication* – all too often ignored, glossed over or not recognized in these non-school-curricular subjects. Teaching is itself an art, and communicating an abstract, creative art requires both verbal and non-verbal skills in transference of *feeling*, as well as information and guidance. If it is worth doing, it is worth doing well.

Teacher training in The Healing School of T'ai-Chi is a minimum of 4 years (usually 5) or as required by an accepted applicant, including theory and written work, and instruction and practice in teaching. Under 30 year is considered too young for the art to be fully comprehended and communicated.

Owing to the outwardly yielding feminine and inwardly firm and spiritual nature of T'ai-chi, there are very few who really have the perception and ability to communicate it *well*, though this situation will improve as we move further into the New Age. It is one of the most subtle of arts, and amongst Westerners will be best communicated through women who have the spiritual and soul-linking with the energies of old China by virtue of their own previous incarnations in that country, always providing they are gifted and fully trained. They are the nearest energy counterpart (with the capacity of the feminine) to the Chinese male teacher of Chinese *cultural* background, of whom there are few remaining today. The Western male, culturally so conditioned in masculine dominance, has generally a longer road to travel to express the subtleties of feminine energy which are characteristic of T'ai-chi form.

Not only the teacher and the student but the art must all develop in accordance with their own indigenous culture and with the Age. T'ai-chi is a living, growing art, expressing and embodying all the processes of change and principles of adapting to circumstances as are more formally presented in the "I Ching". In the Western world, much more specific instruction, intellectual satisfaction, personal concern and inspiration is required than was generally projected for Chinese students of earlier days – whose conception, aims and needs in life were of a different order.

Traditional-style instructors need to be awake to the fact that Westerners are differently polarized by nature compared with the Chinese, and require a different approach. It should be realized that the methods of Chinese masters in the cultural framework and much slower pace of life in old China, are not necessarily at all suitable for Western application. They are often not only out of context but out of date in a world where any teachers or students can avail themselves of more specific and detailed knowledge of processes (including spiritual science). Although respect is essential, it is not necessary for Westerners to bow to Chinese tradition which may or may not be valid, in dress, in study content or in teaching technique. *Methods of presentation and application should not be confused with the knowledge, principle and spirit of any art.*

The criteria should not be what the Chinese or any 'master' said or did, but whether an aspect is in accordance with the spirit and universal principles, and with the facts of both physical and spiritual science as well as with simple common sense. It is not necessary or even desirable for students to dress in Chinese costumes, which was normal dress for the Chinese. We wear what is normal and suitable in our culture. Likewise, we speak in our own language, though occasionally a Chinese instructor (still unassimilated in our culture) requires students to learn the Chinese names of forms (mostly without providing a translation). Addressing an instructor as 'master' also begs the question – how does one then address a female instructor? Master simply means teacher, and it is hardly prudent for anyone to claim to be a master in any higher sense, though others may accord this possibly more out of devotion than knowledge. One should be aware of the very non-T'ai-chi inclinations of some teachers and students who are influenced by superficial glamour and (assumed) 'authenticity' instead of common sense. The keynotes should of course be simplicity (not naivety), integrity, knowledge and inner truth.

Although like other great arts T'ai-chi suffers from superficial projection, it must be remembered that all teachers cannot do otherwise than give according to their own reality and understanding. If a teacher has undertaken reasonable training, this must be respected. On the other hand the art, although created and further developed as a highly sophisticated and potent expression, especially in recent centuries by Buddhist monks, is nevertheless not meant to be the almost fanatically intense and serious thing which it has become in some hands either. In a few schools, rules and rituals virtually create a clique which is little but exotic humbug, and nothing to do with the spirit of T'ai-chi and Tao. Although a fine art and a discipline, T'ai-chi is meant to bring release, enjoyment and inspiration along with the movements of inner growth.

The true teacher is an 'inner' teacher, who has found and is following his own spiritual core, and pointing his students to find and follow theirs. In humility but strength, he is a sign-post and sounding board. A teacher therefore has great responsibility not only as a custodian and transmitter of the art, but through inspiration probably a profound influence upon the well-being and soul-life of the students. He knows that the soul must expand in freedom, and allows the winds of change to move through all his words. He is ever a student of life, of energy and of movement, and applies fine discrimination and wisdom in the evolution and communication of the art in his hands. Chuang Tzu says:

> *In the universe I am but as a small stone or a small tree on a vast mountain. And conscious thus of my own insignificance, what is there of which I can boast?* (Giles trans. Ch.17)

If no fully trained teacher is available, the first discipline is to *wait* until one appears, or until the time is right. This is often the case in country areas, where a group of interested people might obtain a good qualified teacher from the city to visit the area. You can make a valuable start on your own through meditation, and looking honestly at life and yourself, practising soft free-flowing movements which please you, feeling an integral part of your environment and the air you breathe, and by studying the wisdom of Lao Tzu ("Tao Tê Ching"), the Tao and the "I Ching". Remember that the T'ai-chi is much more than the movements.

To study T'ai-chi you may have to travel to another centre, and there are many today who do this for the benefits of good teaching. The forms themselves are not the art, any more than the body is the human being: they are far less than half, but they *are* the essential framework and key upon which everything depends. They must be taught thoroughly – with insight and *meaning*, accuracy and release, or the real art will elude you.

If you initially wish to discover whether the art has anything for you, or to study it properly, you will have the wisdom to watchfully bide your time, and not rush indiscriminately into the first class labelled 'T'ai-chi' that appears, whoever is giving it. It is better to learn half the form or only Part 1 *well*, than to 'get' the whole form in a rushed way. The process is to do with *giving up*, not getting. The modern world suffers much from giddy enthusiasm and 'go-getting', 'forcing the issue' to suit the demands of ego and fashion.

It is worth remembering that one generally gets what one deserves! All good things appear in due season, and thereupon may be received and appreciated in full flavour.

Clothing

Clothing must allow complete freedom of movement, especially around the pelvis and thighs, and be loose or elastically fitting so as to allow a clearly visible body line for instruction. This precludes jeans or skirts. Loose or baggy trousers (not camouflaging the ankles and feet) or tights are very suitable for tuition.

Uniforms are not only unnecessary but not desirable. Apart from Chinese costumes being for Westerners largely an emulation of what was in fact fairly everyday wear to the Chinese, and not so easy to acquire anyway, the drapery of the jackets and trousers camouflages the body line. Uniforms can reduce the adult individual to a formula in a superimposed way, while the art is designed to bring harmony, release and *the natural expression of individual reality* within a self-chosen and self-accepted framework.

Footwear varies in different schools, and could be given more attention. T'ai-chi is not a barefoot exercise, although it may be incidentally so practised, as on the beach or in the garden. The style of forms taught in The Healing

School of T'ai-Chi involves periodically turning on the foot which is carrying the body weight, and so necessitates foot covering: with bare feet or rubber soled shoes, one sticks to the floor and so would inevitably 'pull up' in the middle of the back, instead of remaining relaxed with the base of the spine 'emptied' down. Moreover, students would tend to rely upon the sticking of the feet or the shoe soles, or the hardness of outdoor shoes, to aid balance instead of sensing more their *own* balance; rubber soles also insulate the feet from the earth with which they should be 'breathing', and may lead them to sweat. The wearing of socks or very soft-soled slippers (not ballet shoes) however, enables the student to feel the movements of his own toes, heels and foot muscles in 'breathing' contact with the earth, and can aid the natural adjustment of any foot muscle or bone malalignment.

Practice

Group study and practice is recommended most highly in preference to individual tuition if possible. In moving together, the group and therefore individual energy is developed and shared: the uncertain student may be lifted into greater confidence, while the more able student learns to yield and blend. The healing benefits born of the strength of the group energy generated can be very powerful, and provide experiences of energy and upliftment which would otherwise take maybe years longer to feel, if at all.

The group practice discussed here does not of course refer to classes where students are mostly, if not entirely, diversely engaged in their own exercises. In this situation, energies are not co-ordinated and subordinated into *group* energy. It is not considered by myself to be a satisfactory way of regular teaching for the following reasons:

1. energy movements of individual or groups in the room are in opposition rather than in harmony or unison,

2. necessary and inspirational instruction particularly in non-physical aspects is generally not being given –

   a. because it would require repetition for every student or every small group within the class, or

   b. because not infrequently the teacher does not know enough and can only show the forms.

This is apart from individual practice periods *within* the lesson, as it is very important that students use their own initiative, and can be seen to be doing their own practice and learning, and not merely copying. Students must have confidence, otherwise they cannot or will not practice at home.

Group work is an essential element of the Age we live in – the dawning Age of Aquarius, characterized by the growing feeling for the brotherhood of humanity. Group study in T'ai-chi makes possible the benefits of both group and individual experience, for being a solo exercise, the student in the end is alone with his own energies.

Instruction is normally undertaken indoors, where the student can develop good orientation in space by relating the body to specific directions, and where energy generated can be contained and felt. Individual sensitivity may in this way be heightened and co-ordinated into a strong group energy. Practice in the open air where the vital force is richest is of course highly beneficial for health, especially in a garden or park, and may permit entirely new experiences. On-the-spot standing *ch'i-kung* can be taught and practised outside, but the teaching or practice of T'ai-chi *forms* outside however is best left until the students have come to terms with the structure and direction of the forms to some degree. Otherwise disorientation in space and inaccuracies in direction easily occur, and in any case the energies generated quickly disperse into the air and cannot be felt so well. Early morning practice when the air is clear and the body refreshed is of course ideal, especially in mild or warm weather.

While staying with my friend Ursula Roberts in the south of England, she once watched me practice the T'ai-chi in a little park, and clairvoyantly observed the etheric energy field of a young tree extend across some 50 yards to envelop me as I moved through the forms. A most natural and beautiful sharing of energy through attunement. Although there were other larger trees nearer to me, this one must have 'felt' a particular harmony with my vibrations. As we find tranquillity, we can indeed flow with Nature and become part of her – a wonderful way of cleansing and restoring energies in ways generally unseen but certainly felt. Many readers will know the healing, revitalizing benefits of resting against the trunk of a large oak or pine tree, or wrapping your arms around it to flow with its etheric energy. Relaxing close to a flowing stream or waterfall is also refreshing; if sitting or lying down, point your feet downstream, and imagine the etheric energies flowing through cleansing and strengthening you.

Personal T'ai-chi practice requires a good 3 yards square of space (more for some styles), allowing psychological as well as physical room. It is best undertaken daily in an atmosphere of quiet and inward focus. Any external movements or phenomena in the environment should be accepted with detachment. They might be avoided, but never rejected or shut out, for the discipline is to discover and experience the harmony of the whole.

Relaxing and focussing exercises may be practised beneficially in odd moments as desired or needed, but the forms themselves should never be pressured by time limits. Better to do less and do it well! It should be possible to step beyond time altogether during practice, for otherwise one is not fully aware and not fully in the heart and 'moment' of the forms.

The happiest student is the one who is content to travel along and develop at his own pace, applying himself, but allowing a natural growth within the art without any feeling of pressure or setting of time limits for achievements. As Lao Tzu says

> *By never being an end in himself*
> *He endlessly becomes himself.*[1]

for

> *The least ashamed of men*
> *Goes back if he chooses*
> *He knows both ways,*
> *He starts again.*[2]

Real growth cannot be measured by the instruments of man, but only in terms of the Soul and Spirit. Kahlil Gibran says

> *The soul walks not upon a line,*
> *neither does it grow like a reed.*
> *The soul unfolds itself,*
> *like a lotus of countless petals.*[3]

---

[1] "The Way of Life According to Lao Tzu", Ch.7, Bynner trans.

[2] Ibid., Ch.44.

[3] "The Prophet", of Self-Knowledge, by Kahlil Gibran.

PART II

THE T'AI-CHI EXPERIENCE

Colour & *Clairvoyant Research*

CHAPTER 9
Personal Experiences

Colour, music and movement have all played important parts in my life, and all have clearly manifested throughout many years of spiritual and healing communication through T'ai-chi.

Although showing an early flare for art, and endlessly drawing and painting as a child, my fuller artistic sensitivities were dramatically awakened by a visit to the ballet at the age of 12. The surge of great music, the colour and design of sets and costumes, and the technical and artistic expression through movement: I was awed and inspired! My musical education had formally begun at the age of 11, when I didn't particularly *want* to play the piano; I didn't much want to practice, as at that age my own musicality had yet to awaken. I felt under pressure not to make mistakes, and my teacher was a strange lady! However I *did* want to sing, and I began lessons at the age of 15. The desire to dance was partly frustrated, for my father thought I was 'stage struck' and that the stage was no place for his daughter, and so I had not commenced lessons until I was 14. Four years of dance classes then had to give way to tertiary studies: I had thought of training in commercial art, however I quite unexpectedly (and highly significantly) entered art teacher training instead.

As I had a variety of abilities, there was often a sense of frustration during my teens and twenties wondering who I was and what I was meant to become. Unfortunately, a stale art education at school during the early 50's had left me somewhat stifled and uncreative in many ways – many 'rules', and little attempt to bring out one's own unique ability. I was taught at school, for example, that blue and green do not go together – as if no-one ever looked at nature! Whereas the aliveness of sound and movement seemed so much freer and more immediate, and stirred my soul deeply – the wonderful non-verbal essence of colour and expression in different forms! They seemed far stronger influences for me in those years than art, although art took up a large amount of my time. Music and movement influenced my deeper soul sensitivities, though the values of technical disciplines and the enjoyment of painting, colour and general creative activity in art were greatly appreciated and enjoyed.

Art teaching, writing, amateur and semi-professional theatre continued, and I was always a great reader, but it was music which held me for nearly twenty years, and I eventually satisfied a deep longing for the theatre by spending a number of years with an English opera company. I knew the tremendous power of sound, vibrating both within my own frame and aura, and being immersed in the powerful auric energy of a full company and orchestra. Sound, colour, design and movement – I swam with it all.

All of these experiences were a wonderful preparation for T'ai-chi. Although in the theatre I had (inadvertently) worked with and worked through many of my 'sub-personalities' (elements of past lives), experiencing and expressing much, I had still not found the *complete me*. Although by engagement I was officially a singer, I was often more strongly drawn to the dance and movement aspects of performance, but the root feeling (really an intuitive knowing) was that I was too *individual* in nature to continue indefinitely 'dancing to someone else's tune', to continue to interpret other people's creations. In some way, I needed to get my own hands on the wheel.

Interestingly, T'ai-chi does have a purposefully established but organic framework of forms which one does not alter, a structure at root not unlike the theatre, and I very quickly appreciated (in a simple yet intuitive way at that time) its potential for me as a vehicle. I welcomed this essential limitation as the basis and springboard of experiencing *myself*, and experiencing *for* myself the sheer beauty of a spiritual art with all its depth and philosophy. I had read comparative religion and philosophy since my teens, but the discovery of Tao and its essence in the expression of purity, simplicity, naturalness and acceptance of limitation was such a wonderful release in allowing me to *be myself*. Here was the embodiment, and thus the confirmation, of a philosophy of life which I had always inwardly felt but had never found formulated. Here I could *find me* and *be me*, rather than struggling for acceptance in an alien or artificial reality. Moreover, here was a vehicle by which I could help others to do the same, for the teacher in me has always been very strong.

Here, in T'ai-chi, is the embodiment of all that my body, heart, mind and soul longed for: it *is* music, it *is* colour, it *is* rhythm, it *is* harmony. Not only the practise and discipline, but the inspiring dynamic of its communication as a spiritual and healing art, for it is an expression of wholeness, of completeness, a microcosm of Life. No reaching, no stretching, no proving or justifying. Just Being. Intuitively, I knew that this was my vehicle, to teach not just forms or 'body' (which is *not* the T'ai-chi), but a whole way of life.

Following recognition, my path and commitment were clear. Intuitively I knew that I was right. Early in my studies I became more deeply involved in spiritual training, and through a combination of my own experiences through movement with my developing creative mediumship (the expression of the artist), linked with tapping the higher resources of the Inner Planes of Spirit, I had many deep spiritual experiences and learnt much of T'ai-chi as an art (and of myself) which seems to have been either lost knowledge or yet to be revealed. My early experiences were often of or included colour, for properly aligned (spiritually attuned) practice can awaken the colour senses, as it purifies and balances the *chakras* and auric field as I have described in Part 1. My first impression of colour was green, experienced when moving the arms in a horizontal spreading flow: it awakened the feeling of greenness, with its sense of balance and harmony.

China has a 6,000 year tradition of exercising, both self-defence and therapeutic. Physicians were generally Taoist (aware of nature's rhythms), and taught in little schools attached to their practices, their chief work being preventive medicine: they weren't paid if people got sick! As already described, ease and flow of movement were recognized as essential, involving the whole individual (a microcosm), so that the containing and controlling of energy flow – stemming from harmony of thought and feeling, were the guiding principles.

My spiritual mentors gave me greater details of the 2nd and 3rd Centuries A.D., when there were great developments in the study and practice of therapeutic movements. This was achieved firstly by tapping a past incarnation of mine in China (one of many there) in the 3rd Century when I was a court nobleman's daughter and thus associating with artists and scholars. I was involved in the developments of movement forms, when such women were occasionally engaged for study and taught by Taoist physicians and seers. The seers had much esoteric knowledge including colour and healing. Each movement and gesture, with its mental directive and emotional content, was observed and noted with its effect of the colours produced, purified or transmuted in the auric field, and therefore its effects upon the *chakras* and thus the endocrine glands and whole body response. Images of nature, colour, sound and other forms of inspiration were given, and in both immediate response and in the continuing flow of movement over a period of development, the effects were observed and noted.

We know that each cell and each organ emits its own keynote and corresponding colour vibration. The body is indeed an orchestra of sound and colour. To be 'out of tune' or 'off colour' are true descriptions of disharmony. In my early practice of T'ai-chi, I experienced a number of times what was at that time a wonderful change and charge of energy; sometimes it was uplifting, sometimes just 'different', and sometimes like a colour bath. This was spiritual transfiguration, often by a Chinese personality of the past who wished (and of course was given permission) to share with me his experience and perception, and at other times my own personal Guide (using the vibration of his Chinese life as the poet Li Po), my healing Guide (using his African Ashanti vibration), or another soul energy. I learnt much from it, as I realized that I would only gain by relaxing and surrendering more, though the sight (clairvoyantly) of the transfiguring energy or 'spectre' surprised and even momentarily alarmed one or two students at the time.

A third source of inspiration was via another personality of the 3rd Century whom I had known at that time, who now serves as a bridge of communication for what I have come to call the T'ai-chi Archetype. This is a tremendously powerful energy source, a consciousness formed by a very large number of evolved souls in the Inner Planes embodying the whole wisdom, history, practise and spiritual power of the art. Its spiritual head is given to be Chang San-feng, said to be now a Master in the Inner Planes, who was the initial inspiration of the art of T'ai-chi Ch'uan. This Archetype or source is concerned with growth, not tradition, and will inspire and feed anyone aware of and dedicated to the spiritual, whole art of T'ai-chi who has sufficiently unfolded the intuitive capacity/creative mediumship of the artist. It follows that those communicators who are yet immature in the art (and generally do not realize it) – who are centred in intellective mind control, self-defence and the lower ego of the personality will not recognize or reach this source.

Another important past personality, this time of my own, also emerged in my earth consciousness – an Egyptian trained in the Temple as a seer, serving mainly as an observer in the Halls of Justice, reporting upon the evidence indicated in the aura of the defendant. Many readers may be aware that heightened colour perception frequently marks 'old Egyptian Temple girls', especially those developing spiritual and psychic faculties in creative and healing processes in our present world period; in many cases, those souls (including myself) misused their abilities in the past, and have in succeeding lifetimes been required to resurrect the inner life in order to regain those abilities. This Egyptian personality many years ago came more fully into my present personality quite unexpectedly by transfiguring and speaking through me while I led a meditation within a spiritual teaching session – interestingly, an exercise for gaining better attunement and access to one's Inner Teacher (soul or Higher self), or personal Guide. This energy now remains closer to my 'present' than before in order that her positive qualities of energy and clairvoyant abilities may benefit both me and those whom I serve.

Many of us are receiving the benefits of past life knowledge and experience as we centre our earth consciousness during meditation (including of course the moving meditation of T'ai-chi), and in the flow of our service as teachers, healers and artists. Both Egyptian and Chinese knowledge of colour science and healing, as also of sound and the use of crystals (the latter still in its infancy), are manifesting strongly through the mediumship of many servers in the vanguard of the New Age, and through their inspirational influence the spiritual leaders of tomorrow. (There is much yet to be recovered from Atlantean knowledge of crystals.)

As described in Part 1, the art of T'ai-chi Ch'uan, which emerged as a specific art form from the 11th Century, came to be so-called by the 14th Century. Initially Taoist, and in recent centuries Buddhist seers were largely involved in its esoteric development. Sadly, much of this healing knowledge of the music and colour of life embodied in the design, expression and function of T'ai-chi has been lost, hence the development (a throw-back) of martial applications and terminology. There were those in the employ of the nobility who gained access to the techniques, but not the inner teaching, for it was not understood. Many movements are indeed martial in origin, for Chinese physical education embraced both martial and therapeutic arts, but by the 16th Century the martial orientation had been evolved beyond. The 'whole' art is to 'let go', not to defend. It is to surrender the integrated personality to the directive of the soul and Spirit – for T'ai-chi means *wholeness*.

I have always felt my task as a custodian of T'ai-chi as two-fold: to recover the knowledge which has been lost, and to develop and project the art – so *very* relevant to the needs of our time and materialistic culture, as the spiritually inspiring and healing art which it is. Most projection of T'ai-chi is yet very material and therefore immature, but I know that only the spiritual, healing art can relate to and survive into the New Age. My task, I feel, is to create and project beauty, harmony and truth, and to aid the unfolding of the artist in the individual by creating the environment and flow through which the Light and Sound of the Soul and Spirit may manifest in the Earth.

In all that I have said, I have of course only touched upon the surface, and some elements and healing techniques are not touched upon here at all. As can be understood, the T'ai-chi healing process is a working fundamentally with the whole individual – raising the vibration by energy balancing and alignment, attunement and essential centring through specific practical directives, and through its holistic philosophy and inspirational elements. On the whole, we are not focussing upon curing particular symptoms – the effect of imbalance, nor even upon preventive therapy. We are concerned with raising and balancing the whole vibration. The 'particular symptoms' are worked upon basically through *investing energy in the consciousness of wholeness* – completeness, health and creative enjoyment, raising the consciousness within good body alignment and energy dynamics.

In this book, I present a colour plate showing one of the essential energy streams in the healthy etheric body. It clearly expresses the AUM symbol, and the importance of the Solar Plexus (sun centre or 'psychic brain') as the distribution centre of subtle energy, which can be seen clairvoyantly as vibrations of colour – both as colour streams and auric radiation. In the following pages I will share more of my experiences and clairvoyant research into the auric effects of T'ai-chi practice. To sense or to see into its inner levels of being is to recognize the great beauty of an art, for the outer form is the vehicle for the Inner Light to be made manifest.

CHAPTER 10
Research into the Auric Effects of T'ai-chi

Before proceeding into the observations, I wish to pause to reflect upon a few very relevant factors regarding their import and interpretation.

To appreciate the viewpoint and reality of the observers and their observations which follow in this book, we must remain aware of the limitations of human consciousness and our inclination to adopt and become set in belief structures. We are all of course conditioned by the Age, time, national and racial, social, religious and political culture in which we each have our being, plus our personal life style, economic situation and length of life experience. All these colour our views, even before considering the vast implications of the impact of higher consciousness of both the individual soul and the 'collective unconscious'. We all have our world views of life and reality – all of which are *relative*, not absolute. We are essentially of changing nature in a changing world, and in my view, even the highest human perception is clouded to some degree by the nature of our embodiment in physical matter.

It has always been observable however, that there are many spheres of life in the universe beyond our tangible Earth world, which is but a tiny speck in a vast creation. Countless millions of human spirits continue their existence and evolving on other planes and spheres of life as real as our own, some close to us, others far away from the Earth. Moreover, even as we live this life in our amazingly designed yet heavy earth body, we have our being also in these inner worlds in the form of essential emotional, mental and spiritual human consciousness, and are indeed swimming at this moment *as part of* this vast sea of spiritual life.

Part of the purpose of this section of the book is to bring forward more of the life, activity and reality of these inner worlds into conscious awareness through the meditation of T'ai-chi. It may awaken our perception to the fact that we share our planet and all subtle planes of energy with not only the vast kingdom of humanity (of which only a tiny proportion are ever 'alive' on our world), but with *other* evolutions and kingdoms of nature which do not and have never occupied a dense physical or human form. The realization that these things are *real* is witness to an expansion of consciousness, and the insight that T'ai-chi can indeed be a path to higher consciousness.

Most importantly however, I urge that we must, although enlightened, delighted or inspired by the vision or the evidence, maintain a healthy scepticism as to the *interpretation* placed upon clairvoyant observation, although undoubtedly the more knowledgeable or perceptively advanced reader will certainly understand or infer much from the very modest contribution offered. The psychic faculties of clairvoyance, clairaudience and clairsentience (all people have the last in some degree, though often not crediting it), and most importantly of all, the spiritual (not psychic) faculty of intuition, can provide much knowledge and insight into the nature of life and the whole creative process, hence this aspect of working with T'ai-chi. Mediumship is perhaps the most profoundly *responsible* work to engage in, as although the ability to 'see' is a psychic faculty which must be developed with great care, the spiritual faculty of intuition (a mark of spiritual development) is essential for correct interpretation. Spiritual development is thus indispensable for accurate observation and interpretation.

Quite apart from the necessity of quality mediumship of integrity, observational and personal *interest* as well as capacity varies, as do personal and environmental conditions. Mediumship requires very fine attunement and 'alert passivity' at all times, but owing to the extremely subtle nature of energy alignments, results cannot be ordered or in any way presumed. Ultimately, what is seen or perceived is influenced to some degree by personal *belief*: personal world views and realities and personal experience may shape the material in some way, hence there is no point in engaging the services of mediums who are psychic but not spiritually developed. Properly trained and experienced mediums (not the current 'everybody's channelling') are largely able to step through these problems, and if not will generally decline to serve at that time.

Significantly, Maisie Besant and Ursula Roberts, both co-workers with me for some twenty years, have spent most of their lives associated with Spiritualism (or Spiritism), and both are attuned to seeing spirit Guides or Guardian Spirits (specially trained adepts who have completed the Earth experience), and the many healers, helpers and other spirits on the Astral Plane. They believe certainly in the reality of the souls contacted, as through fifty years of mediumship there are many spirits who were personally known to them in earth life. The reality of genuine contact has long been well proved, but in being spiritually developed women they know very well and have had to work with the wide illusion and deception also coming from that level. Although very attuned to the human kingdom on the Astral Plane, they are nonetheless able to tune in to the elementals (nature spirits) and to the deva or angelic kingdoms, as Eileen Dann does in her observations.

All observers have worked, not surprisingly, within Spiritualism, the one area which welcomes and fruitfully utilizes their abilities. As many readers may be unfamiliar with, or perhaps hold some negative views of this group (the standard of mediumship is variable), it may be useful to note that their basic beliefs are (or were) common to all advanced philosophies and religions, and two are universally held by all Spiritualists – survival of 'death', and the reality of communication with spirits. Many within the Christian Spiritualist Churches in Britain do not believe in reincarnation. However it is very interesting to note that in the early Christian Church, reincarnation was fully accepted, and mediums were engaged for part of their services – as indeed in other early cultures, such as Greece. Unfortunately, politics and tampering with Biblical texts led to much misunderstanding and abuse of mediumship, which unfortunately survives into our own age of materialism. Fortunately this situation is now rapidly changing as old structures give way to the pioneering movements and spiritual awakening of a new Age. My work and this book are part of that movement.

Geoffrey Campbell's observations however barely refer to Guides or helpers, though this was only one occasion of observation. It is significant that he has studied a range of sources of esoteric science and teaching, notably the very valuable but intellectually oriented and shaped material of H.P. Blavatsky (Theosophy) and Alice Bailey. In these sources, genuine communication with the Astral Plane inhabitants, except with adepts or Masters or other exceptional circumstances, is given to be either impossible, or damaging to the evolutionary process of the departed soul. Human forms seen clairvoyantly would thus be overlooked as mere discarded 'shells' or animated thought forms, and not the genuine soul consciousness. To some observers therefore, these forms or figures are ignored rather than studied, though the well trained observer of higher spiritual development can certainly distinguish the real entity from the shell or illusion.

Personally, over twenty years of inter-plane communication has convinced me not only of the reality of the communication possible. I have obtained, to my mind, an incalculable amount of knowledge and sensitivity about the inner worlds and the complexities of the communication process as a whole, not least the effects of thought and feeling, both creative and destructive, upon ourselves and others around us in day to day living. Moreover, much has been usefully and satisfactorily explained regarding both abilities and difficulties within myself and within the students and clients with whom I work and guide. In the teaching of a fine art like T'ai-chi, I found this to be invaluable experience in the training of both my sensitivity as an artist, and of refining my capacity for careful discrimination. The inner life is a world of colour and inner sound, and in working with art, colour, music and meditation in association with T'ai-chi, I find I can facilitate the development of spiritual and psychic faculties of perception for those with the latent ability and the will to do so. It is a beautiful process of evolving one's experience to nearer the source of creation.

The observations and experiences which follow need therefore to be approached with an open mind and heart. Many reading this book will be well acquainted with perception of the inner life, and fully in tune with the spirit and essence of this communication. Others may find some elements very new and challenging. Others again, if strongly conditioned with 'traditional' Chinese cultural realities and belief structures, may find the ideas more difficult to accommodate. If so, I would just repeat what I have stated earlier in this book – that the true Masters of the art of T'ai-chi Ch'uan are interested in *growth* not tradition, except where tradition is still seen to serve a spiritual purpose in a particular time and location. We must remember always that T'ai-chi is about focussing in the Now, not following old and possibly out-moded anachronistic teachings, and about the flow and rhythm of life and the constant requirement to yield and adapt to change in all areas of life.

The evidence of life is growth.

Introduction to Observations

With the students of advanced classes (3rd year +), I have during the late 1980's collected observational evidence of the effects of T'ai-chi practice upon the colours, creation of thought forms and other manifestations within the auric fields of both individuals and groups. For this work I engaged the clairvoyant services of several experienced, spiritually developed mediums who are themselves not T'ai-chi trained.

The qualities of thought and feeling are the key and root of every gesture of expression on the material level, whether or not in conscious awareness. This fact was well known to the Chinese from over 2,000 years of clairvoyant studies of life and movement. The only way to attain healing – wholeness which has been lost, is by balancing, raising and integrating the vibrations of the personality by opening the self to the intuitive/creative levels of the soul consciousness.

To those who 'see' for themselves, the potential of the T'ai-chi experience as a powerful healing process is a practical reality. For those who (believe they) do not see clairvoyantly (and may have clairvoyance without knowing it!), the evidence may be a matter of personal experience of the 'Cosmic Dance', or understood maybe from the observations which I present. Certainly the true healer-teacher can 'see' the vast difference between physically-oriented exercising, and the aspiring or inspired expressions possible for those within spiritually guided healing training. The ability of the student to centre, transmute and release are of course very relevant factors.

Observation 1 – *Viewing from the side of the room.*
Full cycle experienced to the Right.

On the following occasion, four students performed the complete Yang Form cycle of T'ai-chi practice, taking 29 minutes, this pace indicating a slower breathing rhythm than average. The cycle was performed 'to the Right' i.e. at commencement first turning to the right. (It is also practised 'to the Left'.) The students faced the front of the room which is symbolically North (representing the Creative or Source), and moved in normal unison. On entering the room, the observer saw the four students already practising: "What started as a cone of light became a large pyramid filling the room". Significantly, the room is square.

The Form commenced. Maisie Besant wrote: (my comments in brackets)

The four students are placed in square formation within a square room. Circles of an electric blue shade came around Ghislaine. A shaft of light came down like lightning to the right of Peter. I saw the quivering astral body of Ghislaine: she has an emotional or psychic tension (she felt very well but was 4 months pregnant). *Spirit protectors are on guard and she has nothing to fear, although a lot of not very nice thoughts are trying to get in on her.* (These protective spirits are amongst the caring souls working for us on the inner planes – very necessary where spiritual work, healing and service are most evident, since this is where negativity seeks most to disrupt. At this time, Ghislaine had relationship problems at work.)

Orange and mauve lights dart around. A Chinese warrior of the past stands in the midst of the movers (this was during the physically most dynamic section of the forms, where strong movements of releasing energy through the legs as well as arms are powerful movements). *A fountain of rainbow-coloured lights reflect upon the water of a beautiful lake. A crimson flower like a lotus appeared over the heart of Natasha: this indicated a good development of the blending of the inner and outer self – the words come to me "psychic and spiritual coming into unity leads to the heart's desire".* (Natasha has been very conscious of working on this, and recently the changes in her body co-ordination and general integration have noticeably improved.)

A Moses-like figure – long flowing robes and beard with a staff in hand, stood in our midst and was giving blessing to us all (this was near the end of the cycle). *Light was rising up with the hands of Ghislaine. A golden shaft of light was around Peter. A cross of light appeared on the forehead of Giselle* (she was originally Catholic and therefore baptised with the sign of the cross; this symbol remains in the aura throughout life). *A nimbus of light appeared around the head of Peter.*

Observation 2 – *Viewing from the side of the room.*
Full cycle experienced to the Left.
The Candle Dance.

In the following exercise, the five movers were arranged in a circle facing its centre point. This arrangement we normally call the Candle Dance, the movers being connected to the centre or source of light as by a spiritual umbilical cord, as well as the candle being a necessary marker of the physical centre of the group. Moving in a circle in this way has been found to be a very potent means of raising powerful healing energies which can then be used (during or after the practice) for absent healing, or for the healing of someone present by placing them in the vortex of the centre. In a practical sense, the form stepping requires *very* aware adapting to hold the shape of the circle without losing the potency of the expression, but this ability is learnt as part of the experience and training. Other records have since been taken, but although the conditions and energies raised vary, there are many correspondences.

During the opening meditation for centring, Maisie wrote:

Silver blue rising from the centre like a column, and as the group chanted AUM a white angelic form appeared, seeming to hover against a soft lavender background. At this time a small dark cloud formed over Alessandro's head, and within it appeared a child's face (Alessandro's immediate response to this later, was that it might be a brother in spirit who died at 2–3 years old. My thought – it was the incoming soul of his first son born 4 months later).

Later, as the students were more deeply immersed in the essence and flow of the movements, crested waves were seen rolling in with surging foam, submerging all the movers except Rosemary, with whom the water reached only to the waist. (This meaning was immediately understood by all present. Although this group had always been very closely knit, Rosemary had always been somewhat 'apart', finding it difficult to immerse herself and share fully in friendship. The discussion at this point was of great benefit to her.)

Much later, a Chinese mandarin and warrior type of spirit Guide or helper appeared in the centre of the circle, radiating out to each mover. (The students agreed that at that time they felt a very strong bond of harmony and togetherness.)

Our observing medium, Maisie, had no other contact at this period with these students other than this observation of their T'ai-chi practice. After the experience, she gave the following individual readings:

Natasha:

A very earnest young lady with the makings of a good teacher. A misery-me attitude seizes her from time to time, causing her to malfunction with her movements. A stubborn streak is an impediment on the path for her. (Much potential here, but variable application – young, and at times a little easily drawn away from consistent effort. Nevertheless a sincere seeker, who will be able to contribute much valuable service given time and self-discipline.)

Myrna:

Of contemplative nature, but she must guard against absent-minded moments when dealing with material things. A Persian spirit Guide is helping her with meditation, which she finds very difficult to enter into; the Guide wears a long robe and long beard, and a conical headgear. The etheric body has taken over here, which means a self-less attitude is coming more fully into being. Words in glowing light appeared over her head: 'Ye shall go forth in My name, and My conquering power will be with you' – these words coming from the master who has come to her in her meditative life. An immortal, timeless quality is showing, which will help her to overcome all that stands in the way of fulfilling her ambitions.

Ghislaine:

This lady is too 'tied up' with herself, and the etheric energy field was not 'taking over' as it should. She needs to keep more balanced within herself, for the astral body is very shaky. The prayer life at present is very uneven – she needs to meditate more. (In the advanced mover, the T'ai-chi movements 'do themselves': they ride lightly on the etheric momentum generated and guided by the mind. She is perceptive, and normally is able to attain this release very well, but on this occasion and in this period of time she was disturbed by difficulties in her working situation, combined with advancing pregnancy.)

Alessandro:

A silver tree of life appeared behind him: he could use this thought form to enter into meditation. He has an ability to be serene when others around are worked up, but not the capacity to give voice to it. He can be very tongue-tied in any disturbing condition. An eager-hearted, motherly lady in spirit is seen with him. He must not look back to the past with regret, but into the future with renewed hope.

Rosemary:

A great longing for fulfilment with this lady, but so far disappointment only, especially in personal relationships 'You must remember not to wear your heart on your sleeve'. A Sister of Mercy is seen near her, entering into the movement with gusto; she brings a feeling of exaltation.

Very powerful discussions followed around all of these readings, which were valued as being very pertinent, helpful and correct. The sharing of experiences and helping each other is always a part of T'ai-chi training in this School, especially in the 3rd Year and most advanced class.

Observation 3 – *Sensing from the centre of the circle.*
Full cycle to the Right.
The Candle Dance.

It was on this occasion that we placed in the centre not a candle, but for the first time a *person* to sense and record the experience. As normal, the square room was quietly lit, and silent. Being arranged in a circle, the usual symbolic North-facing 'front' for all movers had become the centre point, where Joana McCutcheon now sat with pen and paper, her eyes closed except when writing. The whole cycle was experienced taking 27 minutes, visually like the turning of a wheel, and very beautiful to watch and feel.

Joana wrote: Experiences at the Hub of the Wheel

Butterfly images and diamond-hued many-faceted patternings weaving in and out, the pulsations of energy flashing magenta into blue into purple. Truly a sight of miraculous happenings, a glimpse on the more subtle levels of Being.

The electrical discharges across the room so potent in their force as to alter body chemistry, bringing to the palate changes of taste (to Joana, like sulphur). *Sometimes a whirling like a top spun into space, at other times jewels of many hues in peacock tails, or set in harlequin-like shapes of magenta, blue, red, purple, mauve and violet* (this description corresponded to the physically powerful section where Maisie saw the warrior), *or else just swirling images and colours and electrical discharges of blue weaving through them.*

When the form is good, then so shall be their inner workings. The forms are chan-nelling so much healing energy through these colours. The line of form creates energy, hence colour, movements, and the mind behind the line is the creator. Know you are creating on many levels and are enabling potent healing forces to be released in this way. This is an ancient pattern brought to perfection long ago (i.e. the sacred or cosmic dance, not the present specific T'ai-chi Form itself). *When you do the T'ai-chi you are connecting to the energy forces of the Universe and altering them. All movement does this, but an aware patterning does much more* (a potent point, and referring to the framework of the forms which one does not alter: they repre-sent the Laws of Life within which one must work): *it helps to channel the earth energies in a creative way, thus helping to heal the planet. Be aware also that you are creating sounds of a most harmonious quality when you work in this way.*

T'ai-chi was used in cleansing rites aeons ago (i.e. the essence of T'ai-chi – this style of whole-flowing inspired working through the whole body and psyche). *Use it for peace, for healing yourselves and others.*

Observation 4 – *Sensing from the centre of the circle.*
Full cycle to the Left.
The Candle Dance.

It will be noticed that this is the same exercise as for Observation 3. except that the cycle was performed to the Left direction instead of the Right. Eileen Dann was seated in the centre of the circle, and therefore with most of the movers either to the side or behind her. The use of a small microphone instead of writ-ing enabled her to record in some detail, and she introduces her experiences as follows

I recorded my impressions barely breathing my words into the instrument so as not to disturb the almost electric atmosphere created by them. If my sentences seem a trifle disjointed, it is because I sought to recreate the initial atmosphere, when of course my whispered impressions were brief and to the point.

Eileen wrote: The Candle Dance   (my comments in brackets)

I am sitting in the centre of the circle of waiting figures. The air is now silent as the last breath has died away from the beautifully synchronized AUM sounds which have filled the air with harmony and melody at the start of what is to be an hour of great stillness and peace. This is an Advanced Class; there is a difference between this and an Intermediate which I recently attended. The intonations of the sounds have more depth of tone.

The atmosphere is building up; you can actually feel their thoughts.

Now they start the movements, very co-ordinated. There are four of them and Beverley makes the fifth. Alessandro, Ghislaine, Natasha and Peter. They are turning, and as they turn their arms open. I see the formation of light, joining their hands individually. There is also light coming down from a central point: it is like fine waves of light joining them.

It is so quiet, you can feel the stillness.

(At the time of recording this, I was not aware of what the exercise was meant to represent[1]; I have since been told they call it the Candle Dance.) I recall not being aware of the representation but very aware of colour being evoked – a very pale silvery green, to me representing a sensation of peace. The light around Alessandro has suddenly deepened and become very golden. It hasn't reached the others yet. I have the awareness of candles encircling the moon (see remark above!), *lights, like golden spires. The lights are flickering as they gently move around – it could almost be a candle dance*(!!). *They encircle their right arms and cut the atmosphere – it is as if that is what they are doing* (the impression corresponded to The Stork Cooling its Wings). *You can see a parting, serene and smooth, and this is particularly so with Ghislaine, the symbolic movement of bending down and picking up; it is very beautiful* (– Searching for the Golden Needle at the Bottom of the Sea, and Releasing the Golden Arrow).

Now there is another movement like parting the waves and swimming, very rhythmic. The lights are really flowing now and moving between them like a criss cross of golden cords. I feel the movements like a dance of nature, like conception and birth, regeneration of the self, the throwing away of the old as their knees come up and their hands go out before them. Accepting the new ways and the new path (– the opening of the Release Section in Part 2.[2]).

As they become more involved I see the colours of the Higher Consciousness.

They are still circling. The mauves, magentas, purples and gold are impinging themselves on my mind; I feel they are probably uniting with the Higher Consciousness. I have a picture in my mind of a gentle breeze in a tree with its branches turned towards the ground and the leaves moving gently in the soft wind. They are the trees, their arms are the boughs, the movements made by their fingers are the leaves. I am looking at Ghislaine and Natasha and the expression in their eyes is quite vacant, as though they have self-hypnotized themselves with what they are doing.

I have never really experienced stillness quite like it. It is like being at the bottom of a deep and very still pool. Even the slight movement of their bodies is rhythmic in

---

[1] No representation. Simply following the use of the candle in the centre (not at this time).

[2] Release Section: other teachers generally call this the Kicking Section, but in this school we have no interest in martial applications, as such connotations are not spiritually constructive. We are concerned with root philosophy, symbols and meanings applied and expressed in general life. The movements referred to are powerfully directed released energy, always positive and creative in nature.

unison together. I think they must be drawing to an end as the beam of light is going back towards them.

They are now quiet and standing quite still. (Carrying the Tiger to the Mountain.)

There is a change of awareness in all of them. It is as though they have grown an inch or two. Very, very quiet, deep within themselves. I am in the centre of the ring and they are standing around me. My eyes are now closed in order that I can feel the vibration. Again the energy is building up; it is very, very still.

My crown 'chakra' is opening. The energy is absolutely pouring in. I can feel it travelling down through my body into my legs. I feel very heavy, and yet, conversely, very light. I feel movement starting around me again. The energy is crossing my forehead; I am taking two or three breaths to release it. I can also feel my heart 'chakra' becoming tight. Whereas before the energy was suspended in the area of the ceiling, and the bars of light were going toward the five figures, I am now the focal point. The shaft of light is coming down and engulfing me, and then going out to the four corners like a star with me as the centre; I can feel my solar plexus draining, so I am temporarily shutting it down.

The movement of energy is settling. It is more even now – I feel less pull and more as if I am being 'fed'. I've re-opened my solar plexus, and also allowed the crown 'chakra' to relax.

Vivid colours, a little like a clown's or harlequin's costume, triangles of vivid colour, bright orange, gold, bright green, bright mauve, red; the triangles are standing out very clearly (– Four Corners of the World, also called Jade Girl Works at Shuttles).

The back of my head feels compressed, as though there is a band of energy settling upon it. I have tried to release this, as with my eyes closed I was aware of the energy moving towards me. I've opened my eyes, and found the figures coming nearer; this might explain the feeling of tension at the back of my head. I feel lighter now, and the spiral of energy is going round and round my head. From the top, moving around my body, there is a downward flow toward my feet, spinning very slowly, with me at the centre.

A green cone of light. They have moved out again. I was not conscious of this: I felt they were still moving in, but when I opened my eyes and saw they had moved away I had a sudden change of consciousness myself. The spiral ceased to flow: I must now re-orient myself to new circumstance:– the vibration around me makes me no longer aware of the individual parts of myself. The whole of me seems to be blending together into a oneness. I am no longer green, I am yellow. They are coming in close again. I can feel rather than see it. I am still vibrating; talking into the mike doesn't seem to change it. Opening my eyes I can see they're quite close, and I can feel their auras merging with mine.

Tuning in to Alessandro's there are a lot of dark blues, indigo and magenta. They've done a turn; I 'turned' with them and metaphorically spun around. Natasha's aura is lighter, paler blues and greens like a flag moving gently. Peter's is very similar, a subdued red within it.

I am now conscious of Beverley behind me. Whether she is moving with the figures I am not sure, but I can feel a deeper gold there, also red and deep blue, and I feel it very keenly on my back – for some reason, my own aura isn't merging at the moment. I'm not yet aware of Ghislaine; (pause) I am now aware of her aura: it is rather more a quiet greeny blue, turquoise colour; there is also a deep pink in it. They are moving away again, and retracting their auras more around them. Mine is still moving out; I feel much lighter within myself. I feel the energies moving towards them, instead of coming all into me. Although I'm the centre point or the hub, they're also distributing it around themselves and the four corners of the room.

A movement outside the room caused quite a shadow to go through me. It was only a slight movement, but I think my centres are very open.

They are very close now; I feel quite a tingle on my skin. The triangles of colour which I spoke of before have all merged together. They are rotating more like a Catherine wheel, but very slowly. The colours are all merging, beginning to spin faster; they are right on top of me now. My breathing is blending with theirs. I feel quite sluggish and disinclined to think; I'll just go along with the movement. The effect of the energies has moved into my 'chakras'. The first or base 'chakra' – I can feel a distinct stirring. The pituitary (Crown) is also very active. The energy is flowing between the two quite rapidly, moving around the head to the third eye (the brow 'chakra').

I'm particularly aware of Natasha. Her rainbow arc is moving out toward me. Alessandro's is not.

I've just had a vision of a field of golden corn, dipping and swaying. The five figures remind me of this. They are moving in again, and I'm repeating their breathing pattern. It is as though I'm moving with them, although of course I'm completely stationary. I am so alive and aware. If anybody touched me now I'd jump out of my skin.

A lot of electricity is moving around me. It is like pins and needles in my feet and hands. I'm alive with it. I have the need to keep swallowing; I'm dry. The pins and needles are settling down as they move away again. My eyes now feel very heavy. I feel I could be half out of my body. I'm going to centre myself again.

The strange thing is, I anticipated the sudden swing round they just gave (Riding the Tiger); *I opened my eyes, as if I had received a warning that it was going to happen. I think they are coming very near the end of the cycle. It seems to release the tension. I can feel the break up of energy. The colours are beginning to settle back into blocks. They are much paler now. I can feel a cone settling on my crown 'chakra', and it is moving up and away. The pins and needles have gone. My breathing pattern is again my own. I've become more centred, less aware of what they are doing. They seem to be pulling their auras in around themselves also.* (Carrying the Tiger to the Mountain, Grand Terminus.)

I've opened my eyes. Yes, they are quite still; they've finished the movement. Standing quietly and gently rocking (with the energy). *I feel the energy withdrawing, and from feeling intensely warm, I'm beginning to feel quite cool. The sensation is quite weird. They're turning within themselves, each one again becoming an individual. I'm isolated in the centre, no longer a part, no longer the Hub. I'm very, very small, insignificant, shrunk, and yet very light, clear and cleansed.*

Summary and Introduction to Observations 5 and 6

It is interesting to note that Maisie's 'objective' clairvoyant observations (from the side of the room) were clearly geared according to her regular requirements and work in healing and spiritual guidance, and very valuable in that way (more in the next section). With Joana's more 'subjective' sensing (in the centre), there was a general sense of personal experience of the qualities of the energies and their spiritual import. In the case of Eileen's largely 'subjective' clairvoyance we had a more detailed esoteric and sensitive personal experience recorded. Most clairvoyance is subjective, the medium mentally receiving symbols, pictures and impressions. Objective clairvoyance is rare and more occasional, as it takes a great deal of power.

It will be appreciated that with a group of movers, very detailed and specific recording is indeed more complex and difficult than when the viewer is able to focus full attention upon one person only. As the solo form is in fact the T'ai-chi itself, and the basis of any group working, the two observations which follow of the individual solo practice are essential to complete this section.

These observations by Eileen Dann and Geoffrey Campbell take us more deeply not only into the creation of colours and forms, but the life of the inner planes – of the elemental and deva kingdoms with which we share the infinitely wonderful universe of creation.

With Eileen's record we have the bridging of observation with inspirational and symbolic interpretation. As will be seen, the interpretation flowed very well until the unexpected 'events' of the final sequence of the form: in my own interpretation, the final (13th) sequence symbolizes the final attainment of balance and harmony on all levels, the ultimate integration of the personality with the soul and Spirit. This is evidenced by the unfoldment or vivification of all *chakras*, and thus the moment of final enlightenment is reached – Picking the Lotus Flower, which as a firm and yet fluid 'slap' across the foot initiates and represents the final 'raising of *Kundalini*', the Zen concept of Sudden Enlightenment, and the vision of the Eternal Now followed a moment later by Releasing the Tiger – when one is finally released from 'the wheel of rebirth'.

The reader will find it interesting and rewarding to relate Eileen's experience to that of Geoffrey (especially the last sequence) whom I met again in August 1989, apparently by chance in Melbourne. This was clearly a spiritually inspired meeting, and I had sensed en route to the Bookshop that I was going to meet someone there. He is now free of previous associations wherein he had developed his capacity to observe, record and present exactly such observations as here follow. Although I was tired at the time, we were able to undertake the session in Melbourne before I had to return to London. A second observation for purposes of comparison proved not to be possible in the time available.

It is with particular pleasure and enthusiasm that I share Geoffrey's observations with you. Therein is more evidence of what I have known myself and been teaching for many years, and indeed of what the Chinese saw and knew in evolving the art of movement therapeutics from so many centuries (indeed millennia) ago. My five observers, including Ursula Roberts (see the next section), have not themselves practised the T'ai-chi, and in most cases saw it performed fully for the first time at the time of their observation. Maisie, Joana, Eileen and Ursula have all worked in varying capacities with me and my students, but Geoffrey had had no connection with my students or the T'ai-chi, and I am sure that there will be further studies undertaken in the future when I am living in Melbourne, very possibly with the additional work of a mutual friend and artist.

Having so introduced Observations 5 and 6, I leave the reader now without further interruption to tune in to the experiences of Eileen and Geoffrey, and whatever inspiration and greater awareness they may bring, especially to those who practice the art of T'ai-chi, and to those who may be inspired to undertake this beautiful practice with a good spiritually-based teacher in the future.

Observation 5 – *Viewing from the side of the room.*
Full cycle to the Right.
The solo form.

The following record illustrates the interdependence of life energies, and a measure of how the creative expression of human consciousness can effect other kingdoms of nature. During the experience, the mover is not focussed on any intellectual-level imagery or interpretation of forms, any more than during group practice: it is not necessary or desirable. Rather is the whole awareness upon the creation of harmony, simplicity, clarity and beauty etc., to be in the centre of all things, attaining and maintaining as pure a state of consciousness, of being (emptiness of personality) as is possible, in order to experience and channel the higher vibrations.

Eileen recorded (both subjective and objective):

It is very quiet, very still. She is standing waiting for inspiration, for the energy to spiral towards her. The body is beginning to sway very gently on the spot as the energy begins. It begins to move her body, and to move around the room, and as she moves I am aware that light is moving from her fingers. I am aware of her etheric self outlined round her body. There is that quality of stillness that has nothing to do with being quiet; vague sounds outside in no way distract from what is taking place.

She appears to be making supplication to an unseen force and inviting it to approach her. In her graceful perfect balance she is moving towards me, and I still see the energy that has been surrounding her in the areas where she has moved. As the force field begins to build up I am aware of a golden light. The atmosphere in the room is conducive to what is taking place as it has long been used for spiritual work. Her hands are reminiscent of evoking prayer: it is a real form of supplication to a deity, a dance that is used maybe on a spring evening, asking nature to provide its mantle of gold to the earth, inviting the nature sprites to unfold the beauty of the flowers and the grain. Perfect posture and poise with each movement, studied and yet relaxed ... Other colours are very gradually beginning to mingle with the gold-like fine threads moving about in the atmosphere, becoming entwined with the golden fabric as though nature is moving its colour to the gently weaving form.

She seems to be slowing a little as though the first supplication is complete. The threads of colours are becoming part of the gold. They move into the gold, whereas before they threaded and mingled with it. It is as though she has a fine shawl attached to her wrists, and as she moves her hands the shawl moves and the light moves with it. The colours become more positive. The movements now are involving the sprites: they have joined her and seem to move with her. They are elfin-like figures – butterfly-like with legs, little winged animal creatures but undefined. They form a circle with her as the centre figure as they interweave their colours with hers. It is as though she is lifting the essence of growth from the ground and allowing it to breathe in the air above, drawing the energy of life to her and absorbing it into her 'chakras'.

The ray of light known as the amethyst ray is becoming predominant. The gold is now within the room itself. She is moving within the gold, and the amethyst is blending with it as though a silk scarf has been thrown into the gold and the amethyst colour is absorbed within it. The sprites move into the amethyst, drawing it to themselves, playing with it, weaving patterns with it. Now it is as though she is trying to draw the colour back to her. The sprites are playful as if she is their earth mother; she desires to control them. She is the stronger figure, the earth mother that moves within the field, provides the seed and helps it spring from the ground towards the harvest. She moves the energy away from her as though its clinging threads are impeding her progress. The sprites fall back to sit and watch her, recognizing her strength and dominance over their terrain.

Now it is as though a clearing instead of a room. The harvest yield is growing. An offering is being made to a higher deity – pleasure of the land, fulfilment, eternal growth. She moves within the pattern of colour. We now have a pale rose pink and she pulls this from the ground, still separate from the other colours as of another silken fabric; it changes in shade as she moves her arms. The room is quiet now. There is the same quality of stillness. The movements she makes are barely perceptible to me – very graceful, measured, firmly in control, the earth mother in charge of her terrain and yet conscious of a higher force that directs all, that commands the earth and bids all yield its harvest.

I am drawn again to where the nature sprites are encircling her. They have changed into lights, tiny flickering golden flames, each one about two inches high, a total circle of flame. The flickering has ceased and the flames are steady. She moves in the centre of the ring of flames. It is as though the flame is symbolizing the light within the world that will never be extinguished – that all things are light, nature is light and those that command the growth of nature. The colours are diminishing now, as silver-like threads emanate from her fingers as she moves. The silver represents the light of the moon, the earth quality, that which is stable and drawn to the earth. She bends down, rises and yields her harvest to the moon. The sun has set, the gold has faded and at first became a stronger colour, then faded into the light, and the rays of the silver moon were caught into her fingers.

She is weaving it now to make it part of herself and of the earth on which she stands. The golden flame has much silver quality in it. Small fairy-like creatures seem to tend to the flame to keep it steady. She also has become a flame, an amethyst flame in the centre of her world, part of the earth force of the Age to spread throughout the universe that quality that helps the vibration of Aquarius to steady the earth and bring its richness and promise to fulfilment.

The whole ritual is that of fulfilment, the desire to sow the seed, nurture it and eventually to reap. The offering of the harvest is in her bearing. Leaves of silver are left throughout the atmosphere. She is an amethyst flame in the centre, still moving, still making her offering as she bends and brings that from the earth into the air above (The Snake Goes Down into the Water, and Rises to Attain the 7 Stars). She turns quickly … (Riding the Tiger) … (Picking the Lotus Flower ... Eileen taken by surprise).

In quietness her arms fall to her sides. She brings her feet together. She is at peace within her circle. The golden flames become gently and quietly extinguished; the silent figures of the sprites come and remove them, inclining their heads towards her. The colours gently float into the atmosphere until the amethyst within her settles into its core where it will steadily burn, and the silver and pink merge into the atmosphere as the night continues and all is again at peace.

The mover was Beverley.

Observation 6 – *Viewing from the front of the room.*
Full cycle to the Right.
The solo form.

Geoffrey talked to me afterwards: (My notes in brackets)

The first attunement was that I could see lime green above your head, rose pink to the left, and yellow-white predominating to the right side of the head, and the aura was put into a state of quietude before you commenced.

When you started to move, a kind of nimbus appeared with spears of white and pear-coloured yellow light above your head, and as the movement got under way I saw a flash of blue coming from your throat centre: there were blue rays coming out forward in a V-shape. As you started to turn to the right, there were rays of orange and brown coming from the hands which I believe were the start of the cleansing process; it was then as if your whole body began to shimmer with light. You were getting rid of things that you had collected perhaps during the day, so these colours of orange and brown were perhaps not the purest energy, but they were things that were coming away. Then as you started to sway, I saw a kind of spray of blue and white coming especially from the throat; I felt that towards the start of the movements you were acting quite a bit from the throat, as if you were consciously getting disciplined into those movements, and that effect was coming from there. As it progressed more, I noticed that you seemed to be balanced between some of the lower 'chakras' and I was quite interested in that as well.

*The violet angels or violet devas on the etheric levels seemed to come, and they stood nearby. They didn't seem to make any movements but they stood. I wasn't sure how many of them there were because I was busy watching you, but there were some all around behind you and probably near me as well. They seemed to have an effect that was quietening the surrounding atmosphere. Then I started seeing that there was a deva standing through you – I don't know whether it was your guardian deva or whether it was one that just likes to come when you do T'ai-chi. However the white veils which appeared were as if they were part of the deva, and they were swirling with your hands. I became quite aware of the swirling fluid motion as if you were dressed in veils, very delicate cloth – quite beautiful because the colours were changing quite a bit with the movements, but predominantly I had white – which sometimes means I am not seeing clearly if I see only white, but maybe it was the case that it **was** white.*

I noticed then that the more you started to bend the knees and lower yourself, the energy drifted down to the base of your spine and perhaps into the lower 'chakras', and there was a glowing red energy going down into the earth. At various times during the movements you made specific motions that sent red-orange energy down into the earth (Searching for the Golden Needle; Deep Drive), other times into the sky or other directions (Releasing the Golden Arrow; Releases). Sudden leg kicks with both hands thrusting out as well (Part 2 Releases) created blue and green streams. During the first half of the movements it was as if you were channelling, and it cleansed and washed you from the base of the spine mainly to the throat. It was washing you and flowing very freely through your body – which I found quite surprising, for a lot of people have blockages in various parts of the etheric body. That's what drew me to the meridians which I looked at later on.

I noticed a few startling things at times. For example, you created balls of white and gold with your arms and hands which you then pushed out away from you, and as you did so they rolled away. This often occurred, and when the forward thrust was gentle, but if it was a more definite forward thrust it was as if you sent out a definite stream or streamer of light. Because of the continuity of the movement of your arms and legs, it was very much like streamers and veils of energy coming out. While the outline was like a streamer effect extending out to infinity, there was also the sense that the streamer was sending something else from it, so it wasn't a very simple thing but more of a three or four dimensional entity that was coming out. It was as if it was quilting the sky, an interesting effect, and often wavering and shimmering. At one stage I became aware that you were sending out concentric waves of different colours, and I recorded greens, blues, whites and violets which seemed to be coming from around the centre of the midriff perhaps where the sacral centre is, and even solar plexus sometimes, but it was fairly even and coming out constantly. This was not spherical, but in waves coming out horizontally, which I found interesting.

B: Did this link with horizontal movements like this … ?

Yes, but it was mainly the spinal column that I was observing because the spinal column remains fairly 'fixed' in spite of the other movements.

B: The spine moves in an upright position.

Yes, and because of that, the energy was transverse rather than spherical, so that was interesting. Then at one stage you adjusted your shirt, and it was as if you tore a hole in the fabric you had created: it was very interesting to see that, for everything else was very smooth.

B: I wondered what you noticed at that moment.

It made a tear which was almost a tongue shape, with sharp edges at each end of the tongue.

*A curious thing which I found was that the swirls you constantly created emanated outward **and inward**, and I was observing that astrally more than any other way. For example, there were ribbons of light coming from your third eye, actually more often from other 'chakras', and as you moved the arms the energy was flowing down and out of the arms like a ribbon out to infinity. The origin was from one of the 'chakras', and because you were moving the arms it was as if the emphasis shifted from one 'chakra' to the next in a very smooth kind of way. Sometimes it was being drawn from here, and sometimes here or there, and the light was coming around and through your body, and up and out of your arms. But when I looked **inside** that 'chakra', I could see **the corresponding reflection** of that movement in there: it's like going inside the 'chakra' – like an empty space or a big room, because when you travel in there it widens out, and that's the way space is on the inner planes. You had a corresponding shape going to infinity within as well.*

People tend to look at the aura as being an external, but it is also an internal, and you can take any point of the aura and go inside. With your 'chakras', it's like an infinite pathway that you can follow. It's like space going inward as well, so if you use these 'chakras' as doors, you can say there are pivotal points, and your body is the pivot for the expression of what you are creating with your movements. So I found that it was really interesting to see which 'chakra' did what, because the movement flow between the different chakras' was sometimes linked, sometimes a continuum, but it was going from one 'chakra' to the other, withdrawing energy from one and then adding it to the other in an even kind of way.

So in going inside each 'chakra' you could see the preserved thought form corresponding to that 'chakra', and yet outside in the external you had the combination of all of that being built. It was like constructing a form: if you go right back astrally and have a look at the form, it's as if you have created a very large rose or a large floral kind of shape made of one continuous streamer of light which changes colours. I noticed at one stage that these constant whirls that you had created inward and outward were to me the expression of the soul or Higher Self. I hadn't even latched onto that at the beginning of the attunement, but I'm almost certain that this pivotal expression through the body, and outward as well as inward, is similar to what happens in the soul or causal body (= higher mental vehicle): they say there is a jewel in the centre of it, and from the jewel, light radiates inwards and outwards towards the periphery. So to me it was as if your soul or causal body had been using you as a vehicle of expression – reflecting that light as you did your movement. I found this quite beautiful and quite interesting to think about.

B: Certainly that is what I teach and aim to do – to open the way to the soul body and as far as possible the Higher Self itself, and to do that the lower vehicles have to be open and balanced to allow that expression to come down into creation.

The interesting thing was that I didn't realize it until you were half way through, so perhaps it was a very obvious thing, and my attunement wasn't so hot that I hadn't seen it from the beginning. When it became obvious, I became more and more aware of that as you progressed.

B: Well, you didn't know what you were going to see! I'm thinking about the colours and rose form expressions through the *chakras*, and their creation in the inner levels ... Would you say that you were in essence seeing more the source of the thought and feeling, and then seeing it emerge – taking form outside?

Yes. What made me think of the soul body was that at one stage I was looking at what was controlling the movement. I noted that the mental body was gripping the astral body, and the astral body was gripping the physical-etheric. I sensed that the energy from the third eye was very fixed at times, and from the throat sometimes as well, so that that was the directing thing – that was the stable point. Everything else was fluid in expression, so that even when you pivoted through the lower 'chakras' there was still this red radiation from the third eye, and I recorded blue and violet as well. It would seem to be the stability and controlling factor.

B: Yes, certainly the higher levels should be in charge of the directing of the whole activity, but to what extent do you think that this 'gripping' was partly due to the fatigue which you know I am feeling in the body at this time – gripping as distinct from holding, owing to my slightly strained nervous system in the last couple of days ? (– it was Monday, and I had been teaching all weekend and very busy that morning.) Certainly the 'holding' is an essential part of the directive.

Oh yes, I think it would be gripping no matter what – it's just that if your body elemental fights it, it struggles harder to grip and the effort becomes more obvious.

I said I was interested in the upward and sky thrusts, and it was at this stage that I withdrew and had a good look at the subtle form you were creating. It did go in all directions, this veiled, rose-like appearance that was three dimensional or four dimensional perhaps – because it was different from a rose that you could describe physically. It was extending out perhaps a hundred metres in each direction … Who knows – astral distances you can't measure, but that's what the appearance was to me. It was going down into the earth as much as through the walls and outside (the house), *and I realized that each time you had done this movement or other such movements, you had created a similar rose or pattern which was held somewhere in the background of your aura. It's as if you can leave it here or take it with you, so at one stage I became aware of a kind of universe filled with stars of these patterns you'd created each time you'd had that 'sending out' movement. It was as if you had populated your own solar system inside your aura with the thought forms!*

I was intrigued by the shifting of focus through the arms and legs because they were the vehicles of the energy going through the meridians. I was amazed that when you shifted, the arms were relating very much one to the other a certain balance of energy, like a shifting of energy from one arm to the other as you were moving, and that seemed to determine where the energy went through the body; I couldn't fathom it, I couldn't work out where it was going – I was fascinated, and would like to be able to sit and watch it. (Geoffrey is referring to the constant shifting of energies between polarities of Yin and Yang going on continuously, also through the legs.) *At one stage I felt like standing up and walking over to you so that I could follow where each movement went through – in here, inside your solar plexus, or your sacral or other centres. I was fascinated in the way that the energy was shifting through the body and coming out through the arms – quite a fascinating interplay.*

The cleansing of the blockages was also fascinating. I became aware that you **are** *very purified through these movements, and this is perhaps an ideal way for people who are blocked to release a lot of those blockages in the etheric body. I've never really observed that before. That's why I recognized you in the T.S. Bookshop, because you had that energy and I am used to looking at the devas on the etheric level. Because your etheric body had been released of a lot of those blockages, you are able to move smoothly, otherwise you would have jerkiness in your movements. That was why I could see with you a certain radiation, because other people don't have it. That radiation will never reach the higher 'chakras' in other people, at least not in such a balanced way. So I was impressed with that.*

Yes, and any shaking of the hands sent ripples through the streamer (amused). *At one stage the effect was like an aberration into the whole of the form you had created, and it had far reaching effects in that form. Surprisingly far-reaching, but you had done a lot of good work with those movements: the force effect outward equalled the force effect inward – the thought form outward was equal to the involuted form inward that is inside all 'chakras' as a mirror.*

Then I looked at the guardian deva in flowing veils of white and observed how it had perfect balance in its 'chakras' as well. Often you see devas with an exaggerated 'chakra' through which they mainly function, and they can do so in a purified way and quite safely, whereas if humans enlarge a 'chakra' through over-use, they tend to misuse that energy. This guardian deva had very nicely balanced energies in its 'chakras', and there was a flow going through. Everything was quite beautiful.

B: Where was this deva?

It was standing through your body, moving with your arms, and it had wings that were like veils. Those wings – you know people say that the deva wings are just an auric radiation, but sometimes I think they're not; I think they are a part of the body, because you sometimes see devas which really seem to have wings – almost feathered! This was the case – it was a very gentle veil, and I'm convinced that they were real wings! (amused)

Sometimes when you would thrust your arm or kick your leg, I could see the effects as blue spears extending out into the astral levels.

Towards the end, you clenched your fists and had your arms or wrists crossed (Attaining the Seven Stars), *turned right round* (Riding the Tiger) *and a moment later there was a cracking noise as you lifted your right foot* (Picking the Lotus Flower); *it created a star shape with many edges, a rounded inverted lemniscate. It brought yellow and white like a lightning flash. I don't know how else to explain the zig-zag pattern of lightning – it was emanating from that point in the foot, and then faded. That was an interesting and distinctly different happening.*

As you neared the end of your movement you became enveloped in a triangle of light which was like ... so ... a V-shaped triangle. I realized that it was perhaps to do with the deva as well, for the deva stopped when you stopped, and there was everywhere a calmness. There was a sense of finality to the movement, and this triangle of light seemed to represent something as well, and I sensed that it had something to do with perhaps an archetype, or some kind of form that might have been attached to your personal self somewhere. You know, people talk about there being an archetypal pattern in your mental body, but I saw it as something like a symbol.

Then I became aware at the end when you stopped your movement, that the 'shushumna' channel (of the 3 spinal channels – 'ida, pingala and shushumna') *was visible to me. Maybe it was visible the whole time; before this I was only looking at the spinal column. The spinal column was silvery throughout the whole movement, and when you stopped I became aware that it wasn't just the spinal column but the 'shushumna' – a flow of energy going from bottom to top, and as it neared the top I felt that it came out through the alta major centre at the back of the neck and through the crown centre. I noticed that the 'sutratma' was also very clear, though it wasn't so clear when you started the movement. The 'sutratma' is the silver cord which maintains consciousness between the different bodies, so that when you travel out of your body you are still linked by the 'sutratma' to your body – it's the thread of consciousness that links you to your soul and the Higher Self.*

The 'antahkarana' is something quite distinct from that, and from what I could see it was also stimulated, but I could see more clearly the 'sutratma' or silver cord. The 'sutratma' was connected from the alta major and the crown centre – both channels, but in fact it was probably from one of the glands inside of the head; I could sense that there was a kind of triangle between the third eye, the crown and the alta major. While you were moving it was mainly from the third eye, but predominantly and at the end it was from the alta major and the crown.

B: That is what I would expect.

That was where the stability was: you were directing the movement through the third eye, but in the beginning it started in the throat and moved imperceptibly up to the third eye. Then in fact I wasn't even looking at that because I was interested in watching other movements. I suddenly became aware that your head was 'motionless' almost throughout the expression, and that you were functioning through the third eye; I mean that the head was moving, but it was being 'led' along with the rest of the body, yet it was directing somehow. An interesting thing to observe, because although it was directing, it wasn't outwardly apparent.

B: It was resting on top of the physical.

Yes – it was. That was the odd thing.

B: As in meditation, and this is a moving meditation.

Yes. Then at the end when you settled down again and the aura became quiet, I noticed the colours settling back. I saw the lime green again, and pink and yellow around the head. One can look at other things, but I was only interested in that part. They were devic colours, the lime green and pink, because I've seen a lot of devas and they have those colours, whereas humans tend not to have them so often.

B: That's really wonderful. You have observed so many essential elements of T'ai-chi practice, and evidenced so much of what I have been teaching for many years. I have always felt it to be very important to recover the knowledge and awareness through which this art has been evolved by the Chinese, and although many people do not 'see' what you see in this manner of both objective and subjective clairvoyance, there are many who are well developed in sensitivity through experience who will 'know' these inner realities as we do. That you approached this session with me as a new experience, unacquainted with T'ai-chi, is very significant. It is equally helpful that you have studied spiritual science deeply, so maybe having referred to the *antahkarana* you would clarify its nature as you did the *sutratma*?

The 'antahkarana' is a channel sometimes called the rainbow bridge linking the higher and lower self, and quite often it needs to be built in the sense that in meditation you construct the bridge from the lower to the Higher Self. Eventually you don't need the bridge any more because you have reached the consciousness of the Higher Self. So its purpose is to extend your consciousness, and you'll probably find that the Higher Self is equally building the 'antahkarana' from top to bottom. There will come a point along the way when you will have to understand something of the Higher Self's vibra-

tion and colour or tone, and when that happens you can properly build the 'antahkarana', for many many lifetimes we build it in a very haphazard way. The Higher Self vibrates with a certain colour or tone, a certain sound, and the lower personality self has its own sound, so that when the lower self of colour or sound merges with the higher vibration, the work of building has been completed.

This is why it's good to have a teacher who has the consciousness of the soul or Higher Self, because such a teacher can assist with the building of the 'antahkarana'. They can lead you in the right direction with your meditation so that you construct the 'antahkarana' in the right way – with the right colours that will eventually match with the soul or Higher Self. If however you build along a different line, a different colour, then it's not wasted, but it's not the line of least resistance.

The 'sutratma', the silver cord, is something else. It becomes irradiated or lit up a certain length at different levels of awareness. That is, a person who is conscious on the astral plane while in the waking state will have the 'sutratma' quite brightly lit from the physical brain going up through the astral, but once it hits the mental levels (or perhaps the higher astral level) it becomes dull and harder to see. So – the intensity of the light in the 'sutratma' is related to your degree of consciousness. It's a line of consciousness between you and your soul or Higher Self. When you become illuminated, and see clearly on the astral and mental levels perhaps up to the soul, the 'sutratma' is brilliant all the way. I think there comes a time when the two channels link – the 'antahkarana' and 'sutratma'.

B: Are there any other comments you'd like to share?

Basically I was observing things happening external to you. If I was looking deeply into you, I would perhaps see the reasons why you had taken up T'ai-chi, and maybe the earlier lifetimes – that's possible. It was in the background, but too far away for me to be wandering in there and still keep focus on what you were doing as you moved, so of course that was out of the question.

I felt that your movements were perhaps very closely associated with the devic kingdom. I would hazard a guess and say that you might have incarnated out of that kingdom at some stage (pre-human evolution). I wouldn't have been surprised if there were other devas around imitating the patterns you were creating, because that was the sense I was getting when the other devas appeared around you from the beginning. I thought – Oh we're going to have a formation here! Perhaps I should have had a closer look, but I have noticed that with couples dancing there are devas that create the same astral patterns as they dance in the same room or vicinity. This is something that I'm sure you could evoke quite easily; you could easily attract the devas and they would do those kinds of movements along side of you, and perhaps revel in that.

B: I'm sure that happens.

It is very devic for that to happen, and the T'ai-chi is very similar to a deva class. You know – up in the clouds you have the (more advanced) deva performing certain movements, training the smaller devas of like kind, and they imitate; they manipulate cloud matter or some energy force, and you see it everywhere, not just in the clouds but *in the grasses, and groups of fairies working on blossom trees.*[1] *There is a leader per-forming certain actions with energy, sometimes quite delicate, sometimes quite swift and others imitate and follow. I've seen it even inside the cathedral: I was in St. Paul's Cathedral (Melbourne) after it was closed, privileged to be still in there because I knew the Canon very well, and there was a kind of deva school happening inside the cathedral underneath the nave of the spire. I was quite fascinated to see that because I'd never seen it inside a building. Such things people wouldn't believe! But I think your moving has all the characteristics of a deva, and perhaps this kind of movement comes naturally to you.*

B: Well, I work with the T'ai-chi as a spiritual art, opening the conscious-ness to the soul and higher levels. It's the creative *flow* that really makes the wholeness which is T'ai-chi – that essential characteristic of deva movement. Unfortunately much T'ai-chi today is too occupied with 'being in control', but the only way to attain the real T'ai-chi is by this process of *surrendering* the control and ease of flow of the lower levels to the soul consciousness. So there is the cleansing and the release, but a much higher vibration can be achieved by stepping through the physical working into what I have called the *etheric mo-mentum*, so that the movement *rides* on that momentum. This is definitely a shift of consciousness, so that much of the time one is only just in touch with the outer objective world of consciousness through the awareness of directing the form. Difficult to describe, but it's like looking at the outer world through the third eye. Not as from that point in the body, but rather a highly refined, 'inward' over-all body awareness which is very light and subtle.

One can certainly be aware of overshadowing or transfiguration by an-other consciousness. It can be another soul using a past personality, bridging via the Astral Plane, and I think sometimes a past personality of my own comes to the surface – released to me from my soul body for some particular reason at that time, imbuing me with something of its experience.

I'm sure this is happening as well. Maybe it's not that you are a deva, but that you have simply adopted this style and approach, but it's certainly ingrained, something very deeply programmed into you – like part of your style of being.

B: I know I'm drawing a lot from Chinese lifetimes – not having done T'ai-chi as a practice before, that's not important, but the sense of the Tao, the rhythm, the flow and harmony with all life … There's a lot of Greek in me, and a lot of Egyptian too – both movement and esoteric training, and many other aspects, but certainly those three elements are very clearly evident in my ex-pression, affecting the way I move and perceive.

If you have lived in China you can be very in touch with that kind of energy if you're doing T'ai-chi, or even painting or other dance forms. There's a freedom of flow that exists in the deva kingdom however, that you don't find in normal human beings,

---

[1] He was currently observing much of this in the Botanic Gardens, Melbourne.

and it's part of the nature of a deva to flow and move and have colour, and to communicate through changes of subtlety and colour flow. Everything is free.

B: These things are what I see to be most needed in our culture because we are so linear, so square, so 'posturing' and so geared to getting and having rather than giving. In the flowing of T'ai-chi there can be no postures: it is the continuity of the life force. In the ebb and flow of movement, you become so much a *part of time* in every part of yourself that time virtually ceases to exist during the process of the T'ai-chi cycle. Not if you are too tired and you are more aware of the body heaviness and limitations requiring more effort. This is why the movements are always the same, like a framework, so that you can experience clearly the differences within your changing self.

Yes, and your body is a continuum from lifetime to lifetime in that if you have achieved something of this fluidity in this life-time especially into old age, then you will preserve it and take that quality and ability into another lifetime. Whatever you have now you have built for yourself. (True, but note – this is a general statement on a vast subject; body pliability really stems from adaptability of consciousness, and the abilities of movement may be withdrawn in a particular life for karmic purposes e.g. as difficulty or deformity.)

B: And we continue to build now and create our futures and future forms. Certainly in this life I am able to draw more and more from my past, not a little through the meditative-flow process of T'ai-chi. Part of the purpose of this life for me is to draw together and unify these abilities, and T'ai-chi is a most wonderful vehicle for achieving this – ideal for me, and a necessary rooting practice for grounding my spiritual work. I saw immediately that the art was not just for me, but something which I was to share with others, and through which they too could unify themselves. The person who recommended T'ai-chi to me (and I had never heard of it at that time) was an elderly homeopath, radionic practitioner and clairvoyant who saw the Chinese in me, and foretold that it would "knit my aura". I felt a person of many parts at that stage of my life, and I was rather afraid of failing to work upon that part of me, of developing that part of me that was the most important. I was feeling like a lot of separate fingers, separate abilities, and although I sensed that they were all part of each other, I needed to find the hand to which they belonged. The T'ai-chi proved to be that hand. In working with both the spiritual and inspirational aspects and the physical aspects, there is the possibility through T'ai-chi of this integration of the whole self.

Yes, and I feel that the way for you to develop in T'ai-chi is to continue to increase the depth, because it is only in depth that one finds the inessential human elements.

B: This is the meditation. Each time one performs it, one lives it differently, for all is changing with every moment. Every practice brings a new set of circumstances, a new challenge. Rather like driving: the conditions on the roads and your own personal conditions are always changing; there will be similar situations, and easier and more difficult ones, but never the same ones. Each moment and situation is inevitably unique. During this period today, my nervous energy required extra effort to handle it. At other times I really swim into it, and very immediately feel myself almost lifting out of my body – it is so light, and the form really seems to do itself. One can have quite extraordinary experiences. Today I was aware of other energies there with me, but there are times when it is just a good or very good experience of balancing, refining and emptying the self as I go along, and other times again when I am quite transported – as when transfigured. To have this transporting experience even momentarily at any time during training is such a spur and inspiration, for the release and flow seem so incredibly easy. This *can* happen in very early stages, and it is this that I am steering all students to experience, to discover, if only they can let go and let flow.

Not everyone will discover it.

B: No, but even the little on-the-spot *kung-fu* and *ch'i-kung* exercises can from the first lessons enable that experience to some degree if well taught. The training as a whole process is of course to find that quality and to *sustain* it, to learn to go deeper and deeper within – a possibility intentionally facilitated by the aspect of *length* of the cycle. Nowadays there is a shortened form of T'ai-chi, but the design and balance of energies of the original long form requires the greater depth and sustaining of higher qualities of sensitivity. Through application and flow sustained at length, the finer qualities of this living experience inevitably permeate and transform the quality of life.

Suggestions for further reading:

◆ The Personal Aura – Dora van Gelder Kunz (Quest Books)
◆ Clairvoyant Observations – Geoffrey Hodson (Quest Books)
◆ Handbook of the Aura – Gregory & Treissman (Pilgrims Book Services)
◆ Subtle Body, Essence and Shadow – David Tansley (Thames & Hudson)

A Note About Our Observers

Maisie Besant has served as a medium for fifty years in Britain and also in Canada and Australia, through personal guidance, healing, group training and spiritual talks, with some exceptional abilities unknown to many. Her main teaching Guide, The Teacher now known as Akhenaton, is familiar to many spiritual seekers. She is completing a second book of his teachings and her experiences. (Now 86, she has just taken up T'ai-chi.)

Ursula Roberts has also served as a medium for some fifty years through personal guidance (including auragraphs), healing and group training, and lecturing in many countries, mainly Britain, Europe and Scandinavia. She has written a number of books, including an autobiography, and books of her teaching Guide Ramadahn's wisdom, known to Spiritualists and others around the world.

Eileen Dann has served for many years with personal guidance, healing and group training, mainly in Britain and Ireland, and for some years in Brussels. Her teaching Guide The Master is valued by many seekers, and his teachings are now compiled into a book.

Joana McCutcheon trained in Melbourne, and she shares her abilities through her spiritual ministry with groups and friends. A dedicated spiritual server, she produces beautiful inspirational writing, and as an ex architect she has designed a temple.

Geoffrey Campbell has studied esoteric teachings and trained as a spiritual minister and counsellor in Melbourne. He expresses his own individual form of spiritual service, and has written a book of poetry and clairvoyant observations of angels (devas) and elementals in the Botanic Gardens.

All five people have knowledge and experience of both spiritual and psychic processes, and are of undoubted high integrity. As old soul links, the English women have been for many years working colleagues with me in spiritual training and development work, particularly with my T'ai-chi students.

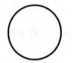

To conclude Part II, Joana is happy for me to share with you the Affirmation which follows overleaf. It would be valuable to learn it as a mantrum, if it appeals to you.

If however you would appreciate a shorter one, I suggest that you might learn that which I wrote in 1977 (see page 136). My groups, and many other groups and friends far and wide, have used it over the years for personal and group harmony and upliftment, so it has acquired quite a power of its own. It is available also as a bookmark from the School.

I AM

I am whole, perfect, vibrant and secure,
the centre and source of my being
eternal and all powerful.

From me radiates the love of humanity,
the security of knowing that I am and always will be.

Within me there resides the jewel of consciousness,
more powerful and more radiant than the sun,
brighter than earthly light and with infinite knowledge.

I must treasure and care for the temporal body garment
of this wonderful jewel
so that it may shine forth in all its glory
for all to know.

I know that I am loved always,
on this plane and beyond, and am secure in that knowledge
never doubting that this love is mine forever.

My mind is serene, for I know that I am eternal spirit,
progressing ever towards the Light, through many lifetimes,
in this and other worlds.

I know that this inner shining light
can brighten the way for all wherever I go.
I will radiate it with love and peace,
knowing that it is from our Divine Creator,
the substance and inspiration of all living matter,
and to which we eternally evolve.

Joana McCutcheon

PART III

STUDENTS' EXPERIENCES

&Further Observations

CHAPTER 11
Discussion of Students' Experiences and Further Observations

Introduction

With more advanced students, the *experience* of T'ai-chi practice is the main focus. When the whole cycle is practised, the students at completion of Grand Terminus remain standing with eyes closed for several minutes according to personal feeling, releasing and integrating the experience. Sometimes they then lie on their backs on the floor (maybe in a circle with feet pointing to the centre), the contrasting horizontal position allowing further emptying and assimilation. On other occasions, following the quiet standing the students have silently proceeded to sit in meditation to observe their physical, emotional and mental conditions, or simply to experience the 'being'. This receptive period is essential for obtaining full benefits.

The sharing of experiences generally follows the quietness after the practice. Although not centred on verbalization, it can, apart from the content, be a valuable exercise in articulation.

The discussions which follow were recorded in London with Advanced classes in May and June 1989.

Experience 1– *Full cycle to the Left, facing North (front).*
Length of participants' experience 3+ years.

Beverley: What was your general experience?

Sharon: I felt really evenly flowing, whereas normally I feel more jaggedy. Sometimes it's OK but then I lose it, and I think probably because you were doing it with us I felt really rounded and flowing. Also I felt the green in the opening meditation very strongly. That helped.

Henrietta: I think the meditation really helped everybody with the atmosphere. I enjoyed it. There was a general feeling, I think from not stopping – of going all the way through (during learning, there are of course many stops). A lot of that was to do with the silence: I like that.

Beverley: Of course. You remember last week – the first time you went right through to the Left? Even though some of you hadn't done it to the Left before, I wanted to leave you to find it in the silence. It went wonderfully well, though there are places where the orientation wasn't clear, but in the flow and silence you can work out quite a lot because you know the form so well to the Right. In being together in a group, there is much that although it wasn't right, you released it and kept going, to adjust it next time.

Martha: I really enjoyed the flow. I felt very 'innocent'. It feels totally different to the Left, and I notice some movements are easier.

Beverley: Are you left handed? Any of you?

Henrietta: Yes I am, and I love it to the Left. I always have done and I would always choose to do it to the Left. I've always learnt with my left. I like it to the Right but it's so much more powerful to the Left.

Beverley: Well as you know it is traditional to turn to the right at the commencement. That's the way it evolved before anyone thought of doing it to the Left. In early times *ch'i-kung* and *kung-fu* were lengthened and then it was thought to reverse them. Mechanically it's obvious that both sides of the body need equal working; all dancers must master technique on both sides as this develops psychological as well as physical symmetry. When we do T'ai-chi to the Left we realize how necessary it is psychologically – an essential aspect of developing mental/emotional balance. Sometimes I've been asked have I ever taught it first to the Left. This would be interesting, but in fact it would be quite impractical because you all come from classes which started at different times. A Left-starting group would be isolated until the advanced level, for they couldn't make up lessons or move to another class as you have had to do at different times.

Henrietta: Also most people are right-handed. I'm sure they must feel to the Right as I do to the Left.

Beverley: Maybe, but the form is very balanced anyway, isn't it. Consider that one takes two years to learn it to the Right originally, and only about a term to reverse it to the Left … The detailed focus and gradual body development inevitably occurs during Right practice, so the two directions will always have a different significance owing to memory and associations. It would take two years to learn to the Left first even if you were left-handed. Also there are people who prefer it to the Left although right-handed.

Sharon: Is there no particular reason why someone prefers it one way?

Beverley: Oh yes, there are always reasons, though mostly they are too subtle for us to know. Certainly there are mechanical reasons – people have particular weaknesses, either congenital or acquired.

Martha: It's about using left or right sides of the brain. I definitely notice the shift in which side of my brain is being used.

Lyn: For me, it's to keep the visualization. As well, it's not so split up in this way of learning it as a whole to the Left.

Beverley: Yes, you know the form and you start doing it to the Left more as a whole, though we repeated Part I at first because it felt strange. Then there are other movements that need extra practice – like the turn to the Bird's

Beak or to Fist Under Elbow, the Twisted Step, the 360° turn, the two Snake movements, and not least Riding the Tiger! They are not just a matter or reorienting but specific practice. But that's a good point – you approach and experience it much more as a whole and it gives you another dimension. I think you were surprised and delighted that it went so well for you.

Lyn: I'm quite delighted about that actually. I thought I'd have to fit it all together again, but it just happened.

Henrietta: I think it depends upon the *confidence* of the individual that they can turn it to the Left. That's all it took – a little while for us to realize that we knew it, and then we could do it.

Beverley: Yes, it's the mirror of the mind working. I think you can see what a loss there is for people who've never *thought* of doing it to the Left. There are so many T'ai-chi students whose instructor hasn't come across it, didn't do it or hadn't passed it on. It's an *obvious* thing to do, and really very necessary for complete development. If you meet a student from elsewhere, ask them if they do full T'ai-chi to the Left.

Manuela: I felt very angular to start with. I was taken by surprise to go through the whole form, but I was amazed how I could manage to do it without much difficulty. I've done it before, but not for some time to the Left, and I was pleased I could remember.

Beverley: Well, it's already there in your computer, isn't it! The archetype is there, and you will have gained from the space in between – since you were last taking classes.

Manuela: I also noticed that the energy was flowing very very well, and almost as if I was getting the strength from Lyn.

Beverley: Mm. You were diagonally opposite one another.

Martha: My heart seemed to be worked much harder moving to the Left.

Beverley: That's something to reflect upon. Keep your head up all the way, and let your heart be more open – let yourself be more 'visible' as a feeling person. Think on that. There is that in you which is hesitant and does not allow you to express fully, for there is sensitivity in you but a hesitation of allowing that to be seen.

Martha: That makes sense.

Lyn: Some of the movements seem stronger on this side. Much easier and more confident. I felt straight and clear – as in …

Henrietta: That's because it's one of those movements which is exactly the same on both sides. It just depends which side you started.

Beverley: Doesn't this illustrate the meaning of directions? You are still using the original North-facing as front for moving to the Left, and it's a bit early yet to turn it to other directions (east, west, south) as you did to the Right; it could 'throw' you. You are used to relating certain movements to a certain direction, and when you turn them around to a different direction you are bringing in a new dimension of consciousness. Take for example The Stork Cooling Its Wings: doing it to the Right, it's the *right* arm – your *consciously strong* side which rises to the side and in a sense partly closing you, psychologically blocking you to the front (North, the Source). This links with the fact that we are by nature *geared* to be right-handed, even if we are left-handed. I have said that left-handedness stems from a past life experience, to do with some action which has been committed through the hand (writing slander, inflicting pain etc.) which the soul wishes strongly to avoid committing again. It's not an important effect to be left-handed, though inconvenient or difficult in some circumstances.

However, when doing T'ai-chi to the Left, that same movement involves the raising of the *left* arm to the side between your body and the front (North). This is not just mirror reversal in a mechanical sense, for the left and right sides, *geared* as they are respectively by the right and left sides of the brain, have different meanings on every level. So no movement is the same 'on the other side'. Remember that the front or North represents the Source, the Tao, and in class the position of the teacher. Since the left side corresponds to the intuitive soul aspects it could be that to raise the *left* arm in that movement feels less obstructed and more 'open' to the Source than the originally learnt right-sided movement. Also, consider that when doing the form to the Right, that particular movement faces West – the Autumn and sunset, whereas in doing the form to the Left one faces East – the Spring and dawn, new life and new beginning.

One could say "Would we be affected if not told this?". The fact is that people are affected by *everything* in and around them in life on every level, most of it not realized. They are subtle – psychological, soul and spiritual aspects. You know that I speak of them to stir your higher consciousness, to awaken greater realization of the inner nature of things – that all outer manifestation stems from the inner levels of Being. The Chinese had a deep feeling for the 5 Directions, much in evidence in the "I Ching". The T'ai-chi movements are intimately related to all these aspects, for it is a callisthenic of high evolution – certainly the form which we have inherited. The whole cycle is deeply symbolic, a spiritual poem expressing the inner and outer order in all creation. T'ai-chi is always a unique experience and instrument for learning, as life is. We are all highly individual and at different stages of awareness in thought, feeling and soul connection.

Well, for my part, I think I enjoyed doing the form with you tonight probably better than at any other time to the Left!

Sharon: I felt you were really enjoying it. You weren't just doing it to show us.

Beverley: When I go through the form with an advanced class it is more useful to you energy-wise if I am really doing 'my thing'. I'm listening to you, but mostly you will be adapting to me as your teacher. I adapt to you when you can't see me. Yes, it was sheer pleasure all the way, and Parting the Wild Horse's Mane really did seem to do itself, a most beautiful movement because it is so gentle and so subtle.

Experience 2 — *Full cycle to the Right, facing North (front).*
Length of experience 3-6 years.
Observer – Ursula Roberts.

Ursula recorded:

When you started the opening meditation there was a beautiful soft blue. During the intoning (sounds in harmony) *there was a marvellous indescribable green which built up slightly into a column of purple which disappeared above. The green was not the one you visualized in the meditation (spring green) but much deeper and greener.*

At first there were waves of light moving across the room, but when you began to move it was flowing the other way like sea waves. Very ethereal. At one juncture during the movements when I was tuned in to it, I felt my chest expanding, though I haven't any chest trouble at all, so I opened my eyes and everyone was doing a chest expansion of some sort, but the energy was coming to me, you see. Then there was a golden ball … but my attention got focussed on Ian, and it was strange – it was almost as if you were becoming transparent and I could see your skeleton (this is etheric vision). *Have you ever had trouble with your bones?* (**Ian** – yes, a broken ankle, recently a hurt back). *Well maybe you need extra calcium to strengthen the whole bone structure. If you've had fractures your body needs extra calcium to rebuild and strengthen … but the scene changed as my attention was drawn to this flowing 'whole group' effect, with energies flowing and separating – streams or ribbons of light energy flowing round from person to person* (**Beverley** – we feel that). *As I sat here quietly I felt myself lifting, and I saw that you were all lifting yourselves up; so there was a general lifting not only of body but the ethereal.*

Towards the end there was a strange 'dust', and I interpreted it that through the movements maybe impurities that were in the body system were being released and given out through the aura like dust. I felt that made sense. When you were doing this (releases – two arms and one leg releasing energy out very strongly) *… there were orange-coloured little balls of fire energy going out. Generally, I tuned in with the whole group, and could feel the changes in the sequences.*

Ghislaine: It's quite interesting about the dust – the words that came were "ashes to ashes, dust to dust", and a definite feeling of letting go. Through that process there is a deeper realization of the beauty of my body, of my personality, a very distinctive awareness that I am not my body or my personality. Quite amazing. I think it's also a continuation of what I did with the homeopath yesterday, and through the breathing and releasing.

Beverley: As if the practice tonight is helping fully to the surface and releasing out what was started yesterday …

Ghislaine: Mmm yes. One of the images that came yesterday when I was at the edge between conscious and unconscious was a beautiful mask. I can't get to like that mask.

Beverley: How did you feel with the group?

Ghislaine: Togetherness. No sense of separation at all.

Beverley: That's very good isn't it. Quite something to achieve. As is clear to Ursula, you all know the form really very well, so it's not a matter of objectively keeping together or remembering. This level is about experiencing.

Elizabeth: The group felt big with you and Ghislaine in it as well. It was quite intimate and so it felt even huge. I have to confess that whenever you do it with us I have a sort of half eye on you for improvements as we go along! I always find that very helpful. There are things I saw in myself I understood, and sometimes they were things you have said and I understood *why* they were like that, like … I watched this a few times and realizing it was a bit crude, I watched and clearly saw that the energy in my hands was only coming up to here – that there was an energy gap, and this hand was adrift and no longer subtle because the energy wasn't coming through properly.

There was a point when I saw you completely Chinese – it almost stopped me in my tracks; it was so Chinese. I've seen you do the form many times, times when it looks like a moving prayer, but it had never struck me that it was a moving Chinese expression particularly. I saw then how much the openness and releasing is to do with full weight shifting, and also when turning to the Bird's Beak – how that knee comes round. You've said "lift the knee" so many times, but I saw that quite clearly. As you've said, we must keep definition in all we're doing (mental clarity) and I realize I don't have definition in that movement. It was seeing that leg move with a quietness that still had a strength to it.

Beverley: It's a matter of having the mind in it.

Elizabeth: Yes, I can see I sacrifice clarity for 'not quite there' softness.

Beverley: Well, it's a long process. At first there is so much of you that is unaware, but by now you notice the parts which are 'dead' because so much has awakened and become 'strung together' in awareness. About the fingertips – you must breathe the energy right down and through the finger tips and allow them to live.

Debbie: To avoid the tension in my neck I was not being precise but too relaxed in order to keep the flow. Because it seemed so slow, my legs felt really bent, and I don't know – I felt really old, feeling like an old woman (she's 21).

Beverley: Maybe it's because of your neck. You felt fine in the group?

Debbie: Oh, yes, it was really nice. Ursula spoke about streams of energy … I was watching you and close to you and could feel the energy waves.

Janys: I think I felt more in unity than before, but not at the beginning. It was more in the 3rd Part that I felt not so separate. What I usually felt about 'people' didn't seem to matter (laughter), as if back to childhood.

Beverley: That's it. You can surrender enough to the group energy of which you are a part. "The sum is greater than its parts".

Ian: A lot of things came up for me. It really seemed like an experience tonight with a lot of changes. Interesting about the bones because I was talking about it before we started. The problem makes me feel very asymmetrical. I was consciously trying to keep the 'squat' in spite of the point of pain. I felt that the group was as unified as it's ever been. I felt like seaweed at one stage.

Ursula: What a good description!

Beverley: Well it's like swimming, having the sense of resistance of the atmosphere, which becomes more tangible as your sensitivity develops.

Ian: I usually feel tingling *ch'i* in the hands at the end, but tonight felt that during the form, that you were controlling the pace from a corner. (Laughter)

Beverley: I guess that's inevitable when I'm doing it with you.

Ian: Once or twice I might have been getting a bit frantic in a quiet way. (Laughter) It slowed me down a bit.

Beverley: In T'ai-chi everything happens in a quiet way. Good description.

Ian: I felt a pulling on the reins a bit. At times it was very good, the form good and the breathing not much of a problem (he has breathing difficulty). A lot of thoughts were coming in, and I was getting caught up in a lot of them. I felt it wasn't causing mistakes or affecting the form much.

Beverley: That's the trap: thoughts come in, but knowing how not to latch onto them. The state of consciousness into which you have shifted allows you to be more open to thoughts coming in. This is where your Soul or Guide can link with you – the opportunity to use that flow will be used. You are doing a highly complex practice, and there is now a certain automation of technique (you all have it in this class) which leaves you free to experience and to witness those thoughts coming in, in a kind of flash – without any frantic element! – to sense whether it is just patter to be ignored or something unusual, significant. In a heightened state of consciousness you can register that; you can't stop and examine it at that time – that would be a major mistake, but it sits up like a little flagpole, so that afterwards when you are free and you reflect, something comes forward like a symbol, or the significance of what was said to you. It's through the flow of energy, the opening and created vortex that you can pick up guidance, and some time afterwards the realization can emerge – maybe when washing the dishes, walking etc., when there is an easy and flowing mental condition.

Carolyn: I really 'got into' my arms tonight – the way they move. A lovely feeling: I never experienced that before. The whole atmosphere of the group was flowing and I could really feel that – it was like wind moving down a branch. It was lovely.

Beverley: Well, it's been a good week. Last night the whole class performed it to the Left surprisingly well, and I could tell them also that my practice with them was the most natural and enjoyable experience I remember to the Left.

Elizabeth, what you were picking up there (the Chinese) may well have been so, because I could feel something of the transfiguration effect that I used to have a lot in my early days of the T'ai-chi experience. There was certainly someone else there right within my aura; it could have been a past personality of my own, because this happens sometimes. You move into that state where you are only partly there – aware of being on the earth plane (directing the form) in that you can see, hear and sense, and although you are very centred and very 'inward' in what appears to be a trance-state, you are not at all losing the 'out there' but heightening your awareness of it in observing it from 'in there'. In expanding your awareness into the soul and spiritual levels, you have the more expanded perception of the world of phenomena and change and its nature of relativity. A condition of being "in the world, but not of it".

Introduction to Experiences 3, 4 and 5

In the following experiences, the students were working in pairs facing each other as in mirror, one practising the form by turning at commencement to the Right, the other turning to the Left. This requires the students to be very proficient on both 'sides' in both technique and adaptability. The solo form requires fine development of centre consciousness, i.e. holding the balance between polarity movements by the characteristically moving centre of gravity through the vertical spine alignment. When working in mirror to each other, the two students must retain their own centredness while developing another centre between each other (see colour plates).

Significantly, to mirror another mover requires adaptability of consciousness to a high degree to allow fine co-ordination and harmony of energies. Having spent years perfecting the form, particularly the basic aspect of correctly proportioned and precise foot placing, the student may initially experience an unwillingness to yield to another's placing and form quality, the ego (albeit in a very subtle way) insisting upon doing it 'my way'. The requirement is to evolve *beyond* the idea of mastering *form* to that of mastering *self*: the form, like all material things, is only 'yours' if you can surrender it, i.e. if you are not attached to it. This practice underlines the fact that the highest achievement and art of T'ai-chi Ch'uan is the ultimate subordination of the material personality aspects with all their earthly motivations (called the Tiger) directed by the mind, to become fully integrated with the Individuality or Soul-Spirit Self. If in the practice one can so raise the consciousness as to express through the movements from the higher intuitive mind (the soul), there can be the finest and most beautiful blending with the soul consciousness of one's partner. This is a very powerful experience.

At commencement the students face each other some six feet apart, eyes closed. They then watch the breathing etc. to centre themselves – firstly creating inner space by breathing out what is past and finished, then visualizing being bathed in the Great White Light, and aware then of breathing in, filling and gently radiating the Light out through the aura; the two auras are visualized blending together, feeling a subtle flow of consciousness linking between the solar plexus, heart and brow *chakras*. The colours frequently visualized or perceived are green/cream-yellow between the solar plexi, green/blue/rose pink between the heart centres, and violet/blue/silver between the brows. This attunement takes only a few moments for the experienced.

The practice then commences as they breathe in unison and allow the form to emerge from idea into expression. As it proceeds, with the form turning in all directions, the mover must perceive the partner's energy and intention through his own aura, especially when facing away, sensing any change or nuance of feeling. At its best it is a marriage of energies, an expression of awareness and acceptance which is compassion and universal love. It is excellent training for marriage – the balancing of polarities in all areas of life relationships which is at the core of our earthly experience.

Experience 3 – *Full cycle in Mirror: Left and Right in pairs.*
Length of experience 3–5 years.

Elizabeth: Although I've felt this at several previous stages, doing Mirrors makes me feel *this* is what T'ai-chi is about, because you are much more acute with yourself, you can't drift in it. The effort of trying to stay in tune with Janys actually forced me to be more in tune with myself. I'm quite amazed at how small and vast at the same time the concentration is. In trying to feel where Janys's momentum is, I concentrate so small it becomes big, and it's not as if it's hard any longer (I know there are mistakes, I can see these things), but in Mirrors one has to let go of it; one has to be able to surrender form.

Beverley: So you have to have it *well* to be able to surrender it.

Elizabeth: It's so subtle that you're not noticing other things, yet what I'm doing with Janys is so big that I can't see Janys or Carolyn …

Janys: I keep thinking– who is this Janys you keep talking about!

Beverley: (laughter) Janys is an external object! (much laughter) What you're saying is an appreciation of the interdependence of polarities: your centre is not a centre *without* the whole periphery. Your vision from your centre only exists by virtue of your becoming more aware of your whole peripheral vision. You understand yourself more by appreciating the multiplicity around you, and that space with all its content takes you back to the 'point' of your own Source. You appreciate that only through contrast. Working with T'ai-chi (or other) form in its increasingly subtle detail, is in a sense only one polarity; the other is the large – the space it occupies, the 'negative' polarity to the accepted positive. The more you perceive the subtle, the more you are in fact expanding your view outwards. People's view outward is limited because their view inward – their inner vision – is so limited. A person who isn't very inward doesn't go very far outward. You see?

For one who can listen and go deeper within, which is going back to the roots of life, the more the consciousness expands to embrace not only the immediate personal friends, relations or whoever, but further and further outwards. The person with universal consciousness feels not merely a part of a family, race or nation but rather a part of the world, the global village, the universal consciousness that sees and accepts everyone as part of himself. The distance that one can see outwards is a reflection, a mirroring of the distance that one has gone within. Makes sense, doesn't it?

Janys: It feels better every time. Although there was the bit we forgot, it's concentratedly together without being a tremendous effort. It feels a very natural togetherness, quite clear. I also find that it's like discovering something that's been there all the time. It feels profound to be doing this – or *beginning* to; just getting an inkling of somebody who was there when I was very young – when I look back ...

Beverley: Yes, the sense of ease that's coming is because you have a good rapport and allowing your auras to blend, and of having your form very well so that you are thinking not so much on an intellectual level but sensing more with the higher level of the mind. You are riding more now on the etheric momentum, moving in space and listening through that space, listening with all your senses fairly well all around your body and the spiritual 'senses' coming in as well. There is an ease of flow in that, whereas on an intellective thinking level it's more rigid and limited. One has to step through that. When you say "we got lost" here or there, then that awareness of the thread, of the moving mental focal point had got lost. Carolyn?

Carolyn: Better. Really nice. I didn't have any doubts this time and we both felt each other – a really nice feeling.

Beverley: I think you feel the benefits of being willing to adapt, to go 'part-way to meet'. But it's one thing to do it with someone you know in the area of studies, and another to do it with someone you don't know. However, the more aware you are of your own soul consciousness, the more aware you are that everyone you meet is a *soul*, and what you are witnessing many times are the struggles of the personality where the soul is not getting through. Where the soul is coming through there will be the linking. So the more you can live from that level, the more you can accept and work with people, even when you recognize that they haven't awakened in the same way. That's wisdom – to accept and not be irritated or annoyed that another person is not 'where you are'. Everyone is where they have allowed themselves to be, according to all their responses in all situations.

Carolyn: So in that kind of situation you have to adapt more.

Beverley: Yes. The other person can't adapt when they don't know where *you* are – though they will usually assume they *do* know! Like the parent and child: the parent has been where the child is, but the child hasn't been where the parent is. If you've *been there*, you can (or should) recognize where the other is. So you don't get subjectively caught up in the behaviour, for you never lose sight of the fact that that one is a *soul*; you understand the personality imperfections and make allowances. Ian?

Ian: It felt miles better, really together that time. One incident which interests me: we got fairly close to the wall, and normally we don't collide, but I was so focussed on … that in doing the Release we collided (laughter).

Beverley: So! You became too specific and lost the holistic.

Carolyn: I didn't feel it as much as a collision in fact, but an unexpected touch. Moving in air, one is particularly sensitive to touch.

Debbie: For me – more relaxed and more together. The bits that I enjoy were 100% better with the other person. I always particularly liked … but it felt even better than usual, and I didn't think it could. When we turned, our minds seemed to do the same thing.

Experience 4 – *Full cycle in Mirror: Left and Right in pairs.*
Length of experience 3–5 years.

Elizabeth: We had to start again, but it was great. I found it fascinating – I know we're doing it opposite each other, but it's actually like a mirror of yourself as well. I felt really easy, obviously having done it more now, we've got more used to it, and I felt it was literally like a mirror when I didn't make it far enough round to the corner facing.

Beverley: Yes, she is another person but at the same time your mirror.

Elizabeth: But I felt very comfortable and wasn't aware of what anyone else was doing (the other pairs working in the room), only us.

Beverley: That's good, because you were the middle pair, and every way you turned you could see another moving. Would you say you have profited from doing it before with Janys – two or three times?

Elizabeth: Yes, because you get the idea of what it's all about. If you're constantly changing people it's as if you're always starting, whereas doing it several times with the same person you can develop it.

Beverley: You have a certain acceptance as a basis. Mind you, you do have to accept *everybody* in due course (laughter). Life is mirrored all the time through different people, but then again a person can mirror you because you know them well; then you can fall into the trap of assuming and anticipating instead of reading what is happening in the *present moment*, and you know that most of the time most people are *not* relating fully to the present, but responding to expectations – projections from the past into the 'future'. Not reading and responding to *what is*, but what they assume or expect. Hence people's fear of being attacked on the street: statistically highly unlikely, but they adopt other people's experience and reality as if it was their own – irrational adopted fears, instead of holding an attitude of creative positiveness – *not* naivety.

Janys: I noticed that we were doing something wrong, and I was doing it *as well*, though I hadn't noticed how it happened. So after that I thought I'd better concentrate and get a grip on myself!

Beverley: Well, one of you was leading the other, and it shows how susceptible one is to another's thinking (or non-thinking!) without realizing it, especially in this art where you endeavour to *blend* all your energies.

Janys: There was such precision in the timing.

Beverley: Yes. More and more you are blending auras, and reading the thought feeling and *intention* of what you are about to do, which communicates itself just a fraction in advance of the movement being performed. This may remind you of Chinese combat challenge: the person who made the first move was considered the loser, since he had not correctly sensed that the other was *not* going to move. You see? The more highly trained one is, the more one links with the movements in the other's *psyche before* they come to expression through form and action.

This is where intuition comes in – a development of higher training, a higher level of tuning and penetrating other energies so that one can sense. It's not a matter of you personally *knowing* someone better to predict what that person may do in that circumstance. In fact, the more spiritually developed people are, the less 'predictable' they are in the ordinary sense. This is a basic reason why the average person, who is generally less able or *thinks* he is (and *is* quite predictable), can be annoyed or envious, and project onto them their own weakness. This happens because the more developed the person, the more their consciousness and being is like a reflecting mirror for whoever regards them. Jesus is a classic example: it is said that "he died for the sins of the world"; I would rather say "he died *because of* the sins of the world" – the darkness, the ignorance, the shadows and lack of love and understanding. They looked upon one such as Jesus, who had such tranquillity of mind and heart, radiating out love rather than taking – for his consciousness and whole auric field was bright and clear like a mirror, not *taking* but just *giving* – living to be, living to give, so that when they looked at him *they saw themselves*, and they didn't like what they saw – for the Light was being shed into their own darkness.

The more you are unfolding your spiritual faculties by following all that you believe is right, is best and beautiful, the more centred and more clearly you are becoming that Christ-like ideal[1], the quieter and more harmonious you are. Because that fight within you is subsiding, other people who still have that fight, that struggle, those shadows, look at you and your tranquillity and like the smooth surface of a clear pool your nature reflects back to them something of themselves. This does not of course mean that they are not *in fact* seeing that weakness in you: the essence of it may well still be present, and can be why you have attracted a particular criticism. But you don't have to be a Buddha or a Jesus to have this capacity: it is part of the karma of more advanced souls – being part of the human race and subject to the lack of understanding of so many of the human race. It is eventually very isolating, for there are fewer others who have that perception, and this must be accepted too. When the ego does not like what it sees (and may secretly admire), it may attempt to pull you down, but you must understand that it is usually *not really you* in fact, but *what you represent*: owing to lack of development, people's perception is limited and earthly, and this distortion (looking out through their own imbalanced auras) leads them to project their weaknesses onto others, and then to try to eradicate them by cutting them down in some way – commonly negative criticism. This is why Jesus said on the cross "forgive them for they know not what they do".

The more advanced a soul you are, the wider your horizons and deeper your perception, hence the greater your responsibilities, and you can recognize those around you who have not reached such a stage. So it is always your task to build and uplift another as part of your own body, never to cut down. And so true compassion is realized, and the fact that one only grows to understanding through experience and the process of distilling the wisdom from it. The enlightened soul does not pull down another because he is spiritually immature, but recognizes the conditions for what they are with detachment, and responds creatively. One can see what the other person is going through, even if they are projecting negatively toward you. If that projection is difficult to take, it's because your own ego is not yet centred.

All this is something to reckon with, because becoming more in tune, more sensitive, does not mean that life becomes more easy or wonderful. Being a good healer for example, doesn't make you immune to disease, be-

---

[1] This is not a matter of following the Christian *religion*, but the unfoldment of Christ-consciousness which is happening all over the world. It is the 'Kingdom' which is coming, and not of this world but born in the consciousness of the advancing soul: *beyond* religious barriers.

cause even if you had no personal karma to work through, there is still the karma of your race, nation and of human nature itself. You have inherited your body from the planet, and thus "all that mankind is heir to". It is naive to think that an advanced soul is immune to human conditions; one may master some (and come to clear understanding of the nature of the others) but not all, for the human condition – though profoundly important in providing conditions and as a tool for experience and learning, is, in being embedded in the material, a very limiting rung of the evolutionary ladder. 'Mastery' in terms of our world depends upon creative acceptance of material limitation and working with it. This is fundamental in T'ai-chi, isn't it: "to yield is to conquer" (Lao Tzu).

So! Life doesn't get easier, but it grows simpler and clearer in essence as you move from being lost in the complex back into the simple. The focus of our working shifts more onto mental and soul levels, the more subtle levels of pain and stress, although a physical condition may also be present … Carolyn, what was your experience?

Carolyn: I enjoyed it. We've done it together before and I could relax along, but it has been better. But I thought it was a bit fast at times, and when I was back to back with you (Ian) I felt uncertain.

Ian: Yes, I felt there was a certain discrepancy of speed, of going faster tonight and a bit ragged. These trousers are a bit tight (not the usual pair), and the effect on the body made me think – my movements were a bit tight tonight.

Beverley: There shouldn't be a discrepancy of speed if you really feel and listen to each other. The more you have been working in T'ai-chi – though things appear to go smoothly, you nevertheless feel all sorts of subtle differences – you are so much more aware of *small* things. That's good! To be aware of what is obvious is easy, but you are aware of things that aren't visible to me.

Debbie: It wasn't very good at the beginning. I think it was because I was doing it with you (amusement), but I tried to let go of it, and I was very aware of how my awareness helped from the beginning – visualizing the connection between us. It was really good: I was trying to send my awareness around us. I wasn't very much in tune with what I was doing though. I felt I didn't know what my hands were doing – I lost them. I think it's because of doing it to the Left. But there were times when I could feel a lot, like when we were facing away in Four Corners: the connection was very strong.

Experience 5 – *Full cycle in Mirror: Left and Right in pairs.*
Length of experience 3–5 years.
Observer – Maisie Besant.

Maisie recorded individual readings and impressions:

Debbie:

Flamelike dartings all round her, an inner impulsiveness to reach out beyond herself was evident. She is an extremely good judge of character, and grasps opportunities quickly. She has the ability, should the occasion arise, to walk away from scenes of turmoil and upset in calmness and composure. There are periods when darkness seems to come in more, but she has determination to rise above it. "The blue of heaven is larger than the cloud" – something happened recently that brought a cloud. She can be very stubborn.

Carolyn:

Blue and silver rays weaving in and out around the head, and ribbons of light rushing down the body. I get the impression of being rather over-cautious and somewhat held in: a restrictive attitude. A tall blonde-haired youth from the past was doing the movements with her; he was very expert with the movements, and helping her. A very small piccaninny girl was with her, imitating the movements and laughing all the time. I could hear the music called "The Solemn Melody" around her.

Beverley: Did you have any sensation of someone helping you, Carolyn? The time is coming when you will. At more extreme times, perhaps doing a demonstration when it's more taxing and more energy being pulled from you, and maybe a little tired and you need something extra. Then you may feel it there. At the other extreme – when you're more deeply in tune and can release and be aware of another energy, which could even be a past personality of your own, or a past Chinese exponent. This is my experience, and that under ordinary conditions one is going along more on one's own momentum.

Maisie: Regarding relating, there was a very good balance between these two – definitely a harmony and flowing peace.

Beverley: Yes, though most of this group haven't been doing Mirrors long.

Chris: Regarding the blonde youth … in a lifetime the body changes shape and features, so would he have died when he was that age?

Maisie: Oh yes. He was quite young, definitely less than 30.

Chris:

The golden rays playing around the head, and the etheric body very much in evidence. A purple light was issuing from the hands. A regal form of an ancient Chinese philosopher-type of man was walking around him, and then withdrawing and coming back again, studying him quite thoughtfully. I saw Chinese writing, and realized that something was being transmitted to him which later on would come into his earthly consciousness as inspired thinking.

Beverley: I've said many times that inspiration comes on flow, and that as you master the form and release your consciousness to ride on the flow the inspiration will come. Interesting that Maisie was sensing the process going on there while you were moving tonight. When you have finished the movements and gone away, at some time that 'material' will come into your consciousness. In other words, it's come into your energies but hasn't descended or revealed itself in your conscious mind. There is an inner realization that comes into consciousness later as inspired thinking.

Chris: I have an interest in writing and I suppose Chinese philosophy as well. Would that be directly connected?

Maisie: This Guide would transmit in Chinese, but because you are now in this Western consciousness you would pick it up in *your* language. You have so obviously *been* Chinese.

Beverley: We attract the old Chinese around here!

Ian:

A phosphorescent light is around the upper part of the body. An inner conflict causes some hesitation at times. A striving after a somewhat hidden ideal which a soul perception will reveal in time. The blue ray of healing is playing around the solar plexus.

Beverley: How did you see the relating between Ian and Chris?

Maisie: There was a rising and falling, like going up on a crest of the wave and then coming right down, but I feel that there was some temperamental attitude in each one that couldn't quite meet the other. You got on very well, then the temperament stepped in, but harmony was achieved.

Beverley: Well, you haven't done Mirrors together before, so it was establishing a new relationship. Just a beginning.

Elizabeth:

An eager enthusiasm trips her up at times. A spirit lady wearing a yashmak is in evidence. There is need for more mind control to develop the capacity for sustained thought and concentration. An opal like mother-of-pearl appeared in the middle of her forehead. She has something of the makings of a rebel, and quite high ideals. A keen awareness of undercurrents of pain and suffering that is with so many weighs on her spirit now and again, but not for long. There's a tendency to be extravert in many ways too. We mustn't give too much, but according to our means – and that means in everything, not just money etc. You must learn to withhold a bit, and not be so much giving out.

Beverley: She does give a lot! And now how did you see the relating between Elizabeth and myself? (I had partnered her because we were an odd number) Was there a difference to when she worked with Debbie?

Maisie: Yes, there was a very strong emerald green colour flowing that circled all around both of you; I felt the flowing waves of energy and light were very good.

Beverley: Carolyn, how did you feel doing Mirrors with Debbie?

Carolyn: I felt a very flowing attunement and very peaceful – no feeling of worries. It didn't feel as strong as usual – thoughts were getting in the way, but otherwise I enjoyed it.

Debbie: It was OK, but I was getting caught up in myself, and made an effort to be more conscious of both of us and it became easier.

Carolyn: The breathing between us seemed quite even; we were riding on the breath at the same pace easily.

Beverley: Now some technical comments! More lift up in the body, both of you. Remember that to relax doesn't mean to collapse! You tend to drop the head during Mirrors. Debbie – breathe more into and through the fingers, and face the body fully into the diagonals, for when turning towards Carolyn you were too self-absorbed and not really relating to her – this matches what you have already indicated.

Chris: I wish I'd asked to do it to the Left instead of the Right.

Beverley: Mm. You had got into it very well by Part 3 – Ian?

Ian: Yes, it might have been better, especially the first bit when I felt quite tense, but there were times when we felt closer together. I had difficulty feeling detached from the situation (Maisie's observing).

Beverley: Ah yes! The ego comes in! You are used to me observing you but this is different, and one can feel apprehensive. There are times when after a drive (martial term 'punch') your back foot is rolling in too soon so that your rooting in that moment is weak, and not fully sustaining the integration with the drive. It's anticipation. And comments for Chris: more full facing into diagonals please, and look also at how you withdraw the energy, and therefore the arms and leg, from the releases ('kicks') – this needs clarifying. Also, move forward more from the pelvis – you were 'leaning over' tonight: keep the shoulders empty and down, and the head up – a stronger lift between the shoulder blades to keep the chest open. Elizabeth, did you enjoy it?

Elizabeth: Yes I enjoyed, though there were fluffs and difficult patches. Having *watched* earlier was interesting, Debbie and Carolyn having very different qualities. Everyone was quite unique and looked effortless, though I know it takes a lot of concentration to do that. Debbie's centre of gravity is quite low which makes her very stable, and when I was doing it with her I felt that the more I lowered *my* centre of gravity, the more it became automatic, and then we were in the same timing.

Beverley: Yes. Now it's up to you to meet together and develop that attunement. Class time is too limited to give much more than the keys, each partner being a totally different being. Now my comments to you Elizabeth: *relate more to diagonals* – there needs to be more consciousness there – and you know this is so for several of you: the four corners are not as obvious as the four sides, and tend to be given the glance rather than the full attention. I felt when I was moving with you that you were whipping away! I wanted to be more fully 'in it' with you, but you were leading me on much of the time before I had completed the statement. This was partly I think because you need to allow yourself to breathe *out* more completely, and allow the breath to come in again when it is ready, but I know it was partly also a little anxiety because you were doing it with *me* …

Remember that although I am your guide – your 'sounding-board' and 'sign-post' on the way, I am another soul and personality to whom to relate. Whoever the other person, respect them, but don't be diffident. Remember that the task is to find your own reality, and to express it creatively in harmony. Be modest but confident in finding and being your *own self*.

Well – time is gone, and that is a positive note on which to finish. Thank you Maisie for sharing with us.

Experience 6 – *Full cycle in Bi-symmetry, square formation*
2 moving to the Right, 2 to the Left.
Length of experience 3+ years.

Another, and probably the most interesting and popular of the variations we call Bi-symmetry. Like the Candle Dance it is a group exercise. The Candle Dance is a *circle* formation with the movers, from five to maybe seven or eight, facing the centre point and everyone moving in the same direction like a wheel. Four movers may also be placed in a *square*, and all perform the T'ai-chi in the normal way either to the Right or to the Left: this is still a wheel-like formation but in being in a square is reminiscent of a swastika.

Bi-symmetry practice however is based upon the *square* and four people facing inwards, and is a particularly interesting arrangement with two people opposite each other moving to the Left, and the other two facing opposite each other moving to the Right.

In Figure A, the standing positions at commencement show that those who will move to the Left are opposite each other, as are those to move to the Right. In Figure B, the interesting nature of this variation becomes clear when movement commences. At first the movers approach each other at right angles, and we are aware of Relationship 1.

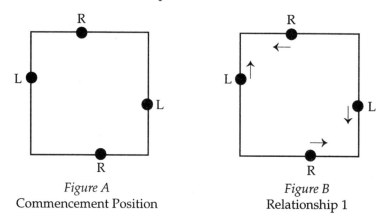

Figure A
Commencement Position

Figure B
Relationship 1

Shortly afterwards they face outwards as in Figure C, then across the diagonal or 'corner' as in Figure D. Further travelling takes them to face and move in the other direction, as in Figure E where the development of Relationship 2 is appreciated. At the end of Part 1, shown in Figure F – Carrying the Tiger to the Mountain, all four movers have travelled across and are facing inwards and relating to each other in unity which we may call Relationship 3.

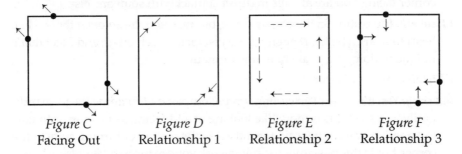

| Figure C | Figure D | Figure E | Figure F |
| Facing Out | Relationship 1 | Relationship 2 | Relationship 3 |

The interesting, indeed fascinating pattern of weaving the form and the dynamic of changing relationships amongst the movers, is an absorbing experience and very beautiful to watch (see colour plates).

Elizabeth: When we do this, I often feel it's like a castle or Norman keep, so strong and square. I've usually done it before with Chris or a male energy, but today (all women) it felt so 'fine', as if we were making gossamer rather than bricks!

Beverley: I would agree with that (she and I were moving adjacent to each other). There was a little too much wafting with you at first: I'd like a little more linear quality and directness – it was getting a little emotional. The key to this is in the carriage of your head. In this press-back movement you were leaning your head in anticipation of the next gesture, and not fully relating to me while I was still facing you. It was a little introverted, and not conscious enough of our relationship.

Elizabeth: Yes that's true. Probably holding the baby too much! (she had just returned from assisting at the birth of a T'ai-chi friend's child)

Beverley: Your movements needed a clearer line. Make sure your pelvis turns fully to the corner, so that you fully acknowledge that position … I seem to remember saying this before! However you were picking up my corrective signals very well! I appreciate your description of the strong and square Norman keep.

Elizabeth: Yes. I'm aware of these angles today and realize that the angles and angle-facings are so important – turning to face another person in the corners.

Beverley: It strikes me that this exercise really brings out the meaning of your corner facings. When learning and performing the form in the normal way, one is fairly clearly aware and able to relate to front, back and parallels (left and right sides), but it's always taken everyone some time to fully "face your corners" as I often say, those 'corners' within yourself which you would avoid or ignore. In Bi-symmetry one is more conscious of corner form movements because you 'meet' (face) a person there, and so it has a more particular purpose and potency. When you turn away from the corner again – to the parallel or outwards of the square, you are more 'on your own' again; in corner facing you are always in direct contact with someone else.

Elizabeth: Interesting in the corner-work, because you are so open there – like heart to heart. The heart energies are just facing each other, and I feel that's unique to doing the T'ai-chi in this formation.

Ghislaine: Yes that's true.

Beverley: Yes, it's more of an *opening away*. Compared with doing the form ordinarily as a solo, this is more like looking at and facing self – more intimate. Put another way, in the solo form there is the feeling of turning *away* to the corner, but in this bi-symmetric framework you are turning *towards* and *opening up* both to yourself and to another person as well, rather than opening yourself up in a quiet little corner unnoticed. Interestingly, we do this spreading open of the arms (swimming) and roll back movement so many times facing the corner …

Elizabeth: When doing Cloud Hands I was facing straight across the square to Ghislaine, and I'd never fully seen that relationship before either. In Mirrors we would both be travelling in the same direction although facing each other, but in Bi-symmetry facing across the square, we were both going to the Right and so travelling in opposite directions.

Ghislaine: I think I was very aware of the flow, receiving from one side and then giving it out to the other, giving a sense of circle, like rounding the square. Although the framework was square, the flow of energy was definitely the give and take of roundness. There was more of the sense of spinning …

Elizabeth: Spinning the gossamer … I felt that too. When we did Cloud Hands in Part 2, I felt we were Chinese ladies doing a dance. I felt it really strongly because we were all so 'in step' doing it, very together. That was an unusual image for me, but it was a very dainty energy at that point, very fine and sensitive.

Beverley: That particular movement *is* very refined as you find how it works. The side-stepping is so quietly neat, and the gentle turning in the upper body and circling of the arms and hands is all very simple and contained.

Ghislaine: Very etheric – the quality of the clouds: you can't touch them, you can't grasp them.

Elizabeth: It's true. I've watched clouds, and I remember lying in the garden wearing glasses which filter out the glare so that you can really see what happens with the sun and clouds. The clouds don't just sit there but drift apart from each other all the time, drifting away or into themselves.

Beverley: One can understand why the Chinese Taoists used the clouds as a symbol of the Tao – mysterious, ethereal, ever changing.

Janys: What strikes me about Cloud Hands is that in Bi-symmetry you are such a long way from most people in the room when you do it. The opposite person is across the room from you, yet in feeling you can be very close.

Beverley: So as with other variations it is important to be carefully positioned at the beginning.

Ghislaine: If we end up too far away from each other there is the feeling of remoteness, of losing contact.

Beverley: Yes, that's true, but the link must be there in consciousness, and the holding effect of the pattern is always there.

Elizabeth: It's interesting as well to be in your own space – not too close. It's as interesting to *be* more isolated as it is to be close!

Beverley: In this exercise the four movers remain very much individuals, for the direct relating is for shorter periods of time within the length of the form – at one time to this person on your left, at another to the one on your right. The mirroring is still there whether close together or more distant. The times of being quite close can be quite powerful, but part of the exercise is maintaining that contact of awareness, even at a distance.

Elizabeth: It's different from Mirrors, where there is intensity of focus with just one other person all the time. In Bi-symmetry, when one turns and meets another person 'in the corner' it's like a joyful experience!

Beverley: In turning to the corner there is to me a sense of revelation, of meeting the unexpected in a way. It's not the same sort of confrontation and potency that you seem to feel in Mirrors. Your attention changes periodically from one partner to the other, and for this reason in particular I feel that Bi-symmetry is the variation that is most like everyday life. In both variations the other person is like another part of yourself, but also reflecting yourself: you feel very conscious of the other's energy, but at the same time very much the reflection of yourself – and this is strong stuff!

Ghislaine: A matter of facing up to it.

Janys: There's no getting away from it!

Beverley: In working in a four, there is a certain relaxation in the attention being divided as the focus shifts from one to another. It allows more a sense of ease and requires adaptation and agility. Also, there is the factor that *all the time* the *expression itself* is mirroring our response to everything and everybody around us. It will be good when you can take the sense of ease you feel in Bi-symmetry into Mirrors.

Janys: I felt a very nice sense of anaesthetic afterwards. Very softly part of every-thing. Not a precise thing. At the end when I lay down on the floor, I had that very soft feeling which is lovely, and I haven't had it since last term. I could see too what you meant about continuity of energy movement through the wrists and hands. Also, I enjoyed those bits when I turned and faced Ghislaine.

Ghislaine: I felt a peace, a constant adaptation from one energy (person) to another. It was very absorbing to keep your own boat aflow. Like waves but of different qualities coming. Constantly building, melting. I felt something of the quality of joy, which opens me and makes me feel soft. I feel that this experience for me tonight will be long remembered.

Elizabeth: Interesting that the floor can feel soft, lying down on it I didn't really register it was the floor. (It is parquet)

Beverley: You were allowing your body to flow with the floor.

Elizabeth: I did feel that. Even at the end when I was standing with eyes closed the energy felt like gossamer, but strong and fine. The play had built this fine energy, and when I sat and lay down afterwards I had felt the vastness of things – a really lovely 'place' to be.

Ghislaine: I felt the weaving. Each separate colour, separate thread or fibre just disappears into the pattern. I really had something of the melting qualities, and the idea of weaving has just come to me. We were all different colours, different individuals, but somehow we came together and melted; individu-alities not separate any more. There was a real healing and coming together. I think there is something very personal in it. With the experience of to-night, I am aware of that.

Beverley: Do you feel there are any other characteristics of Bi-symmetry ?

Elizabeth: I feel it's more like the world. It's the most 'material' form of our working together. Quite earthy to do this compared to the other variations. It's the strength and power of the manifest world.

Beverley: Being held together in weaving a pattern – a co-operative.

Elizabeth: For me it's strongly to do with the fact that when we are at 'corners' to each other, we are open to each other.

Ghislaine: It's in some way like bringing the Candle Dance (circle working) and mirrors ('parallel' working) together, because Candle Dance is more the group energy, coming together and surrendering to the whole. We have that in Bi-symmetry, but we also have the more individual relationships with one person or the other, and the personal opening out in this way is very important – how much are you willing to open or not open? But this is not as potent or direct as in Mirrors'.

Beverley: Bi-symmetry seems to offer the best of both worlds, doesn't it – the blending of different elements. What about the Candle Dance, when you all move in the same direction and are all spokes of one wheel?

Elizabeth: I feel that the Candle Dance is completely cosmic! Not this Earth at all to me! We give ourselves up as part of that wheel. It's too difficult to really evaluate what you are doing – especially the first time we did it.

Beverley: It came off very well indeed the first time you did it.

Ghislaine: It was magic! (Ghislaine first did it some years before)

Elizabeth: Yes! Whereas Bi-symmetry seems to say that 'the Earth is OK' – with bodies and people and all! Again I think of those corners, for the opening to another energy at the corners is gentler and somehow more 'human' than mirroring directly.

Beverley: Well, you know that it's not to last all that long (much laughter). Also, there are the times of moving away, facing more outside the group when you are not immediately involved with some particular relationship. You are in your own aloneness when facing outwards, though still following your path in life according to the rhythms of nature – knowing yourself to be still part of the overall swim and pattern of life.

Ghislaine: And in the quiet you are able to assimilate and integrate that experience. This Bi-symmetry seems to me to provide more the range of human experience, with its changing and varied kinds of relating. But there is also the sustaining: there is not just relating once, but the coming back, meeting again – building a relationship with a person as a process of growth, of unfolding, and not too much at once.

Beverley: Yes – we have the repeated meeting and withdrawing in Mirrors, but there is only the one energy to return to which does require staying power and becomes a very powerful experience. It's more perhaps like dealing with a specific problem or developing a particular talent by repeatedly investing energy into it – good creative energy.

In Bi-symmetry we have the greater variety of opportunities for adapting to changing energies or circumstances.

What riches the T'ai-chi has given us to discover!

Let us give the last words to Lao Tzu, that soul (or whoever it really was) from whom we have drawn so much inspiration and insight into the nature of life, the spirit and essence of the Tao, and its embodiment in the beautiful art of T'ai-chi Ch'uan.

Before creation a presence existed,
Self-contained, complete,
Formless, voiceless, mateless,
Changeless,
Which yet pervaded itself
With unending motherhood.
Though there can be no name for it,
I have called it 'the way of life'.
Perhaps I should have called it 'the fullness of life',
Since fullness implies widening into space,
Implies still further widening,
Implies widening until the circle is whole.
In this sense
The way of life is fulfilled,
Heaven is fulfilled,
Earth fulfilled
And a fit man also is fulfilled
These are the four amplitudes of the universe
And a fit man is one of them:
Man rounding the way of earth,
Earth rounding the way of heaven,
Heaven rounding the way of life
Till the circle is full.

Lao Tzu

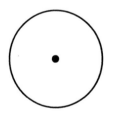

From "The Way of Life According to Lao Tzu", translated by Witter Bynner, Chapter 25.

CHAPTER 12
Conclusions – Today and Tomorrow

Considering the scope of our subject, all that I have shared I feel to be modest and introductory. My thoughts and the inner teaching which I know lies behind and within them, I hope may inspire further inquiry, and deeper understanding and respect for the spirit and essence of T'ai-chi. Ultimately it is a personal living experience, which like all the arts and the Tao itself, is beyond the power of words.

Those who have long travelled the T'ai-chi Way, whatever the form and instruction, I trust will feel my thoughts and identify with the inner verities in their own way. Those who are just approaching or have just begun, I would hope – as with my own students – to inspire the best which the art has to offer. Whatever our viewpoint however, it is best to remain open-hearted. What we understand and will know tomorrow depends upon how we see and conduct today. We should reject nothing either – especially unfamiliar views and teachings, but seek to understand if not to accept, and to be in harmony if not to agree.

My object in bringing out something of the inner essence and meaning of T'ai-chi is, apart from being my own reality, a recognition and requirement of the Age. We live in a material world where personality has been so much divorced from Spirit. The yielding and receptive nature of the feminine, embodied in creative expression through the use of the higher intuitive mind, has been suppressed by the dominance of the intellective and reasoning masculine nature embodied in materialism. We suffer from over-stimulation, emotional pressures of competition and ambition, and uncertainty of standards due to the speed of change in a technological age. The human being and his need of the spiritual and feminine elements has come close to being left behind by his machines, and almost forgotten. So follows frustration. Lack of concentration and self-knowledge, incorrect body usage, and difficulty in relating to others – in short inadequate response to life.

Yet the Divine Plan is being fulfilled. Even as we witness and are involved in the turbulence and breaking down of the old order, we are experiencing the energies and birth pangs of a *new* age. In recent decades, a great belt of spiritual energy has been built around the earth, and those who are in tune will be able to link in and move forward with strength into this new era of spiritual evolution. The revival of the spirit and essence of T'ai-chi is part of that Plan.

By building and strengthening the bridge to a life of higher awareness, T'ai-chi can loosen the hold of the material. Through its fundamental structure of sinking and spreading the weight – the acceptance of Mother Earth, and the lightness of carriage and aspiration to the Spiritual (instead of earthly) Father, we have a framework for the recovery of inner and outer balance, and the discovery and expression of one's own unique Individuality. As a complete art, it has the keys to the broadening and rounding of the whole 'too linear', top-heavy Western personality.

Those who have undertaken training in T'ai-chi with instructors trained in the East, or in traditional methods and therefore the traditional Chinese conception of *ch'i*, will have noted a rather different conception of energy and its use discussed in this book. I make no claim (nor wish to) to following or in any way necessarily adhering to traditional views, unless those methods and views correspond to my own knowledge and experience as of continuing validity and universal verity. In my experience, the Chinese conception of *ch'i* seems limited as generally projected, in acupuncture as well as T'ai-chi.

There is every reason for, and possibility of improving this situation by the study and application of spiritual science, including esoteric anatomy. The oft expressed "developing of *ch'i*" seems little understood except in a physical perspective (including conscious mental), for it is evidently projected as far more concerned with self-preservation than complete inner balance and *letting go of the ego*. Martial usage and connotations have no place in the New Age now dawning. T'ai-chi must be adapted to Western world conditions and our spiritual requirements in the current age. Any real masters of the art, and most certainly all those who look back from the higher planes of spirit, are concerned not with tradition but *development*.

Those who have an understanding of the full essence of T'ai-chi are very rare, and rarely write. It involves so much inner knowing which is beyond the power of words. Yet it is they who are sowing the seeds. As already discussed, because of the outwardly feminine and inwardly spiritual nature of T'ai-chi there are few who have the perception and ability to communicate its inner reality in our culture.

To write on the *nature* and *meaning* of T'ai-chi is of far more value – in my estimation – to everyone, both students and non-students, than the apparently endless production of manuals (and now videos) of what to do and how to do it. Why, as in any other movement art, people cannot be left to go and see it for themselves and study T'ai-chi in the natural (and necessary) way, is not difficult to divine. It seems easy with a conveniently 'set' framework of Form (though varying in different schools and teachers, a fact which many people do not at first realize), to fill paper with form descriptions and photographs (interesting to a degree but quite inadequate), and to publish at a time of popular press. Certainly it is valid as a creative expression on the part of the presenter, but it is serving self more than serving the art or the people. Often the reason given is to serve those in outlying areas. I refused two publishers to write such a book. What information is given in many such books is largely repetitive of previous texts, and although all books have value in communicating an *idea* of *some* kind of T'ai-chi, information of the presumed history of the art is most often (innocently) incorrect. There is either lack of real knowledge or insight, or lack of courage to express it.

Much of the real history of T'ai-chi has never been written, chiefly owing to lack of authentic information. As we have seen, the art has come to public notice and the Western world by way of the Chinese nobility rather than the monasteries, so that much of it has become projected in self-defence terms.

Little has been written in any detail on correct body alignment, breathing and relaxation through meditation in T'ai-chi in the English language. Almost nothing is available on its symbolism related to life, particularly our present-day culture, or the T'ai-chi philosophy in action in the forms: this is very fertile ground for writing, for it can bring new perspectives and much needed inspiration.

In a few areas today however, where intuition is flowering and admitting an inflow of spiritual perception, there *are* refreshing and welcome insights unfolding, and it is to be hoped that they will be shared. Much of great value can also be written about T'ai-chi related to the many walks of life, to soul and spiritual growth, and to the other arts, for new harmonies of rhythm, music and colour are already entering into its expression. If we are to relate to T'ai-chi adequately in and through our own culture and our own Age, we *need* these broadening perspectives.

The art of T'ai-chi is indeed a cultural masterpiece – 'the cream of Chinese culture'. Its inherent philosophy speaks of Universal Truth. It is our task to find The Way, and express it in our own terms.

As part of my own Way, I wrote during the 1970's the Affirmation that follows, which over the years has been used or adopted by hundreds of my students, and travelled far and wide. As an inner well-spring and focus for thought, it has acquired a power from which you may like to draw, and into which you may contribute something of your own energy.

I would like to take this opportunity to share it with you, my readers. May it bring you strength, joy and inner peace.

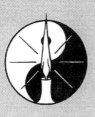

I am the Living Spirit.

I am at peace and in harmony
with all life and with all vibrations.

In all my Being I grow ever upwards
in the Light and Beauty of Truth.

In all that I do,
at all times and in all ways,
may the Living Spirit be manifest
in and through me,
that I may be a living light
in the service of others.

Peace.

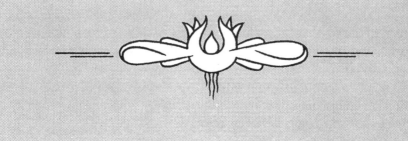

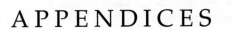

APPENDICES

APPENDIX A
The Values of T'ai-chi Ch'uan

As indicated in the text, these values are extraordinarily comprehensive. If linked with common sense nutritional care, daily practice may lead to a long, active and healthy progress through life.

These values may be summarized as follows:
1. How to *combat illness* of mind and body,
2. How to build the skill to *maintain health*,
3. How to *increase* resources and potentialities,
4. How to *reach understanding* of the inner nature,
5. How to *apply the will*.

In physical terms:

1. co-ordinates physical body
2. relaxes whole body
3. stimulates circulation of blood, oxygen, lymph
4. deepens breathing, therefore better respiration, purer blood
5. strengthens heart and lungs
6. loosens joints, increase flexibility
7. strengthens legs to support body
8. improves stamina
9. finds centre of balance
10. tones up skin
11. improves vocal, visual and aural efficiency
12. prevents illness (unless karmic)
13. prevents freak injuries (unless karmic)
14. contain energy, control energy
15. massages internal organs
16. improves sleep
17. very valuable for pregnant woman, mother and child.

... etc.

In more subtle terms:

1. integrates whole system
2. teaches self-control
3. develops patience, perseverance
4. calms and steadies emotions
5. gives confidence
6. focusses mind, concentration
7. improves memory
8. mental alertness – avoids habit
9. makes one face reality/faults
10. teaches adaptability
11. aids orientation in space
12. develops awareness – physical, emotional, mental, spiritual
13. heightens perception – vivifies *chakras* and psychic body naturally
14. provides general release
15. develops rhythm and musicality
16. facilitates creative expression
17. develops healing abilities
18. promotes clarity and simplicity
19. promotes appreciation of arts and cultural refinement – music, poetry, dance, art, sculpture etc.
20. promotes balanced development of the unborn child.

... etc.

APPENDIX B

The Five Animals Movements

This delightful 4-minute cycle of 12 *ch'i-kung* exercises, taught periodically in my School, is an excellent example of the old traditional natural therapeutics.

I inherited the cycle in 1980 from John Lee, who had inherited a wide range of therapeutic teachings and traditional exercises, including the 14 Meridian Movements which he also taught me. As much of the breathing-movement alignment of the 5 Animals cycle had been lost, I completed it as a continuously flowing *ch'i-kung*.

In identifying with birds and animals and their natural movements and expressions (as we find in other early cultures), these exercises aimed to create and maintain a state of integrated naturalness and flow, as they assisted the release of the personality ego through creative play. In earliest times, people would roll, tumble and play even lying on the floor, with accompanying noises! As indicated by their delightful names, the movements are full of character, providing most enjoyable and stimulating contrasts of psychological attention, colour and mood, as well as their obvious physical dynamics. One might call them 'being meditations'.

The cycle is accessible to people of all ages, of particular appeal to children, and to the child within every adult. It is a very balanced general *kung-fu*, and participants are encouraged to let go and make noises – e.g. the Monkey Eating the Peach, or the Tiger Roaring at the Cliff Face, and allow themselves to identify with and *become* the animal or bird.

The Cycle

Unity Prayer
 – *opening attunement, lifting, balancing, centring*
1. Phoenix Flaps its Wings
 – *light, lifting arms*
2. White Monkey Eats a Peach
 – *bending, spreading, mischievous*
3. Fierce Tiger Emerges from the Cave
 – *crouching, pressing, curious*
4. Bear Stretches his Limbs
 – *firm up/down, claps, wrist-turning*
5. Young Tiger Plays in the Mountains
 – *side extending, playful*
6. Bear Hangs from the Branch
 – *up/down stretching, bend, arm spread*

7. Monkey Curls and Kicks his Limbs
    – balancing, wrist/ankle turns

8. Tiger Roars at the Cliff Face
    – firm, fierce, dramatic

9. Deer Plays in the Early Morning Sun
    – light, lifting, elegant

10. Crane Soars
    – light, full circling

11. White Monkey Picks the Stars
    – firm, sideways leg-slaps

12. Bear Stamps
    – firm up/down, heel thump

    Unity Prayer
    – closing attunement and symmetry

At conclusion, stand quietly with eyes closed to aid assimilation.

A five minute meditation is very beneficial.

It is recommended to read the novel "Monkey" by Wu Ch'eng-en (16th Cent, translated by Arthur Waley), a popular and delightful classic and allegory: it tells the story of the fall and redemption of Man, represented by Monkey who embodies all the weaknesses of human (earthly) nature. Exercise 2 refers to the Peach of Immortality stolen by Monkey in the Heavenly Peach Garden.

The 5 Animals cycle is taught periodically.

APPENDIX C
Exercises

Exercise 1 – Spine Release

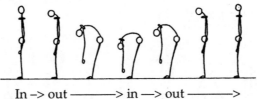

In –> out ————–> in —-> out ————–>

a. Stand with feet slightly apart, arms hanging, head poised over the spine, and face forward.

b. Breathe in to start, allowing the breath to flow up to the head and down to the base of the spine.

c. At the top of the inbreath, let the head lift and tip gently forward.

d. On the flow of the outbreath let the head continue to fall forward followed immediately and consecutively by the cervical vertebrae (neck), dorsal spine and shoulders, and lumbar spine (small of back) – all on the one outbreath, until the upper body hangs right down (the legs are loosely straight).

e. While hanging downwards, loosely and gently move the head to assist full neck release.

f. On the next inbreath, smoothly raise the upper body in an unfolding motion, keeping the tail down and drawing up and back first the lumbar spine.

g. When the shoulders rise above the hip level and begin to drop, change to the outbreath to raise the upper torso and shoulders, draw the neck up and back, and finally the head. This outbreath allows the shoulders to sink as the neck and head rise. The lift through the spine should be clear and strong.

h. When fully upright, stand still for a moment or two with the head lightly poised to allow the blood to settle.

Images

1. Visualize the breath as a cleansing, refreshing green, turquoise or peaceful blue stream of life, of water, of energy etc., washing right through the head and spine, and at the end flowing down and out on the outbreath through the top of the head like a fountain. If your nervous system is strained, a violet stream of light is helpful. If cold or tired, breathe in orange or golden yellow through your feet and legs into the body, or a clear yellow for general cleansing. Clear radiant white light energy is always safe and beneficial.

2. Feel as flexible as a young blade of grass or reed, moving on the 'inner breeze', and visualizing green.

3. Imagine the vertebrae as bright pearly beads loosely threaded on a string.

Values

Opens the spinal links via the breathing and natural body weight, especially of the neck and lumbar regions, thus releasing neck tensions by drawing out the muscles, loosens the shoulders, circulates more blood around the head, nourishes the nervous system, and strengthens the back muscles.

Exercise 2 – The Joy of Life

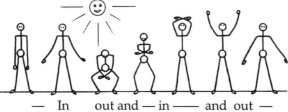

— In   out and — in ——— and out —

a. Stand with heels about 1 foot apart, toes turned out 45°.

b. Breathe in to start, letting the arms rise loosely to the sides.

c. On the outbreath, bend the knees (pointing outwards over the toes) and swing the hands downwards towards the floor, imaginatively scooping and gathering, allowing the wrists to cross as if embracing. Allow the head to drop, keep the tail down, and do not sink so low that you are squatting.

d. On the next inbreath, lift up in the legs and body, crossed arms rising past the chest and heart centre, and on upwards, opening out above the head like a flower unfolding.

e. On the next outbreath, bend the knees outwards again as you sink and gather again, arms swinging down in a circle.

Images

1. A growing flower emerging from the earth, opening to the sun.

2. Washing and bathing in the waters of life.

3. Gathering the fruits of your life and sharing them.

4. Flowing through the continuous cycle of nature – birth, growth, death and rebirth – the circular movement of renewal.

5. The gathering movement may represent experiences, the crossing of the arms the nurturing and integrating of them, and the opening out of the arms the releasing/putting into practice.

6. Express your movements with imaginary music.

Notes

Just let yourself go – express yourself and *feel good!* Let the arms flow in full circles, keep the neck loose, and allow the head to look up and down with the arms; feel every part of yourself. Repeat 4 – 5 times.

Values

Physically – opens the hip and shoulder joints, loosens the spine, strengthens back and legs, opens the thorax and improves balance. Mentally and emotionally – allows positive release and expression. Stirs *all* energies into rhythmic motion. Spiritually – the more you release the self, the more the soul and Higher Self can speak through and to you, and the more whole you feel and become.

Exercise 3 – Circular Roll

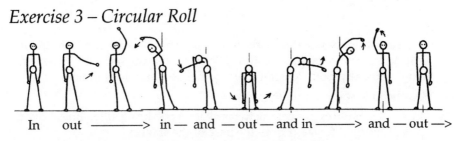

In   out ————> in — and — out — and in ————> and — out —>

a. Stand with feet slightly apart, arms hanging to your sides.
b. Head poised over the spine, breathe in to start.
c. On the outbreath, the Right arm lifts out sideways to above the head, shoulders still relaxed and level.
d. On the next inbreath, lift and lean the body and Right arm over to the Left and *slightly forward*, allowing the Right side and lower back to 'yawn' open.
e. Breathe out slowly, allowing the Right arm and body continue downwards on the curve until the whole body – head and *both* arms, and hanging forward loosely. NB as the body tips over towards the Left, the Right arm must be allowed to *drop loosely* from the shoulder.
f. Continue the rolling movement slowly over to the Right side, lifting the Left arm and head (in alignment), 'yawning' open the Left side of the body.
g. When the Left arm is above the head (shoulders level), breathe out to lower it gently down to the Left side again.
h. Repeat the movement, commencing with the Left arm.

Notes

The tail must be kept down, and non-travelling arm hanging loose. Keep head in line with spinal flow at all times, and when lifting the neck and head at the end – keep the back of the neck lengthened and move slowly and carefully. Repeat a second time if you wish.

Values

Releases any cramped feeling around the waist after long sitting or standing, eases the lumbar back region, opens shoulder joints and loosens the whole length of the spine, gently 'using' all back and shoulder muscles, oxygenates the body and improves general circulation.

Exercise 4 – Standing and Sitting

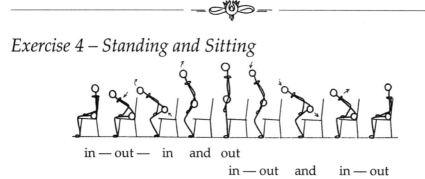

in — out — in   and   out
                in — out   and   in — out

a. Sit on an ordinary wooden chair, feet apart near the chairlegs, with thighs a little apart. The hands are resting lightly on the thighs, with upper arms hanging loosely from the shoulders, spine erect and head in line.

b. Breathe in to start.

c. On the next outbreath, keeping the neck long and head still in line above the spine, lean right forward from the base of the spine.

d. On the next inbreath and moving continuously, imagine being drawn forward and upward by a thread by the crown of the head – which keeps the spine and neck full length, and eventually lifts the buttocks off the chair. Continue the movement to standing position on this inbreath, drawn all the way up through the head – without pulling in the back or crumpling the neck! Then breathe out to stand erect.

e. Breathe in to start (continuing straight on).

f. On the outbreath, keeping head and spine still in line, allow the full length of head-to-spine to lean forward as you bend the knees, imagining being drawn down by the base of the spine towards the chair. When the buttocks touch the chair, breathe in to draw head and torso upright via the head.

Notes

No pulling in of the back to lift the buttocks off the chair or put them down again; *no* throwing back of the head or crumpling the neck at any time. Shoulders remain at rest throughout, relaxed and loose.

Values

Integrates body movement smoothly with the breath, facilitating continuous flowing movement; keeps centre of gravity in the right place; exercises the body in good alignment, removing causes of tension in the neck and lower back; strengthens the legs – intended to support body weight.

See what you can do for yourself. Have a good critical and objective look at yourself naked in front of a mirror, full length if possible. Remember that no-one's body is perfectly symmetrical: we are all inevitably a *little* out of balance, but this 'little' should be minimal. Ask for advice from someone close to you if you are interested and concerned. Major adjustments require an expert. If you suffer a lot from headaches, or fatigue which is difficult to account for, you should obtain expert advice and help from a well qualified practitioner.

APPENDIX D
Taoist Meditative Breathing

Abstract meditation was practised by early Taoists, who achieved transcendental wisdom. Connected with meditation were breathing techniques which we usually associate with Yoga, used by Taoist monks for the attainment of Tao. There is ample evidence that the Chinese had developed complex breathing techniques long before the advent of Indian influence, and Lao Tzu himself advocated breathing exercises for purification and concentration. The Indian and Chinese Yoga systems are very different, owing to different philosophical background development. There is however a striking resemblance to the Taoist technique and goal in meditative breathing, in the Sutra on Breathing by the Buddhist monk Tao-an (312 – 285 B.C.). It can be seen that Buddhist and Taoist techniques and goals are essentially the same in meditative breathing.

Sources of the Taoist System of Meditative Breathing

"I Ching"

Theories of the 5 Elements

Yin and Yang Principles

Lao Tzu and Chuang Tzu

and later –   Chinese alchemy, numerology etc.

Macrocosmic / Microcosmic view of Man – the universe contained within the individual.

The inner force centres (*chakras*) of the body were known in China before 1000 B.C., for they were closely linked with Acupuncture. Meditative breathing and the inner centres are mentioned in medical works of the 4rd and 3th Centuries B.C.; voluntary and involuntary circulations are described, and a whole chapter deals with the circulation of the breath and its relation to the fluctuations between Yin and Yang principles.

The Inner Elixir School

The earliest Taoist texts on meditative breathing (– no mention of Indian practices) were published in the 2nd Century A.D.: "Meditation on Identity and Unity" by Wei Pe-yang. It speaks of using the forces of Heaven and Earth to compound an inner elixir of immortality. The Inner Elixir School theory is that 3 principles are compounded:

1. *Ching* (essence)
2. *Ch'i* (breath)
3. *Shên* (spirit).

Each principle consists of 2 aspects –

a. material (visible)
b. primordial (invisible).

Ching (essence)

The material force = *sperm, the body vitality* maintaining energy and life, but this is not complete without understanding its primordial aspect: through *breathing* one draws in this Cosmic force to be compounded.

Ch'i (breathe)

The material force = *diaphragmatic breathing* of the beginner at meditation, but this is not complete without developing *embryonic breathing*, the primordial aspect from which one draws in this Cosmic force to be compounded.

Shên (spirit)

The material force = *ordinary consciousness* – one's senses, perceptions, thoughts, feelings from birth, and the *spiritual consciousness* from pre-birth, but these are not complete without *primordial spiritual consciousness* which is revealed through meditation.

The Object of Taoist Meditative Breathing

The object of Taoist meditative breathing was to unify the 2 elements of one's original nature which were supposed to have been divided at birth:

    (a) *ming* – life or destiny (the material), which could be lengthened through *deep breathing*.

    (b) *hsing* – spiritual consciousness, which could be awakened to enlightenment through *concentration on nothingness*.

The union of these 2 is the attainment of Oneness, or Non-being, and so *ming* and *hsing* are basic concepts in the theory of Taoist breathing. Through meditation, one's personality self is subordinated to become integrated with The 10,000 Things: the Macrocosm. Just as movement is the fundamental unifying element in the universe (Macrocosm), *so breathing is the unifying element bringing about Oneness in Man (microcosm).*

This idea of *Man as a microcosmic universe* is basic to Taoist meditation. The physical functions and organs of the body have cosmic analogies upon which the breathing system is based. The earliest Taoist analogy system dates from the 2nd Century B.C.

Taoist Breathing Technique

Slow, deep and rhythmic. There are 2 main courses along which the breath or *ch'i* is directed by the mind, which together form a complete circulation through the body.

    (a) **The Lesser Heavenly Circulation** – the involuntary descending course. On the Yin *inbreath*, air is sent down from the imaginary heart centre (the Chinese centre of thought) in the chest, to the region of the navel and kidney (the centre of the Earth). This begins as diaphragmatic breathing, but graduates to the sending of a mental idea along with the movement of the breath.

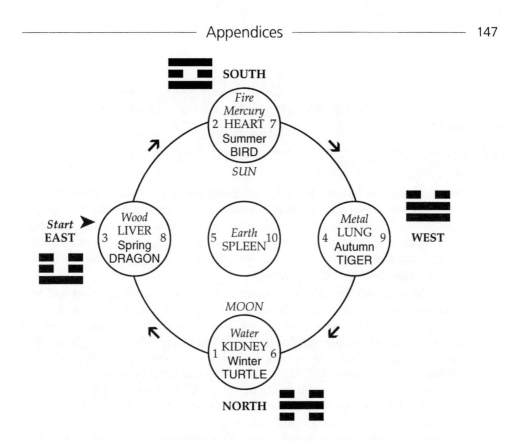

(b) **The Grand Heavenly Circulation** – the voluntary ascending course. On the Yang *outbreath*, the idea of the breath or *ch'i* is sent from the coccyx up the spine to the head, forward and downward through the face to the top lip. The Lesser Heavenly Circulation will then continue on the inbreath as air is drawn in. The Grand Heavenly Circulation is thus known as the union of Heaven and Earth.

The breath does not literally travel of course: it is a pathway travelled by the *mind*. With practice, one can send the idea or *ch'i* to any part of the body at will, and feel it (e.g. as heat) move along the path. This is said only to exist in a state of deep inner awareness, of no-thought (such as we endeavour to develop in the T'ai-chi). When one achieves true quiescence, the "heavenly radiance" emerges. The whole basis of breathing as a meditation is self-realization. It is important to note that the chief requirement is for the meditator to understand the principles philosophically, or the exercises may be only a hindrance.

Modern neurology would probably explain these circulations as a very high psychic concentration in the sympathetic nerve fibres, which creates a stimulus resulting in electrical current. Scientifically speaking, this procedure stimulates the nervous system.

APPENDIX E

The Healing School of T'ai-Chi
Melbourne

A Summary of Studies

The School offers holistic training, emphasizing that harmony of outward expression flows from an inner state of mental-emotional focus and balance permeated by Spiritual reality. It is directed as guidance and training for those seeking or endeavouring to follow a spiritual path or growth programme. Self-acceptance, building creative relationships and healing group energies are important aspects of the School's life.

The complete Yang Form is taught in detail (structure, meaning and feeling) over two years or more (right side practice), comprising 13 sequences within 3 Parts. The cycle takes between 27 and 30 minutes to perform, the movements riding specifically on the flow of breath as a *ch'i-kung*. The form style is subtle and refined. The 3rd year involves left side study (reversal of the right side cycle), mirrors (partnering), and other variations for four or more people developing finer sensitivity and attunement, and allowing assimilation of experience for health and growth. A Teachers' Certificate training is available for accepted applicants; training is individual, requiring a minimum of 4 years, and includes detailed theory as well as practical studies in all essential aspects of the art and its effective communication.

The Five Animals' Movements are offered periodically, and are available to non-School students. A delightful 4-minute therapeutic cycle riding on the breath (*ch'i-kung*), open to all ages, it is based upon the natural expressions of the tiger, monkey, deer, bear, crane and phoenix.

Study commences with breathing-movement (*ch'i-kung*), general workout exercises (*kung-fu*), attunements and T'ai-chi preparation forms in the 1st Term. The Form cycle itself is commenced at the beginning of the 2nd Term. Relevant Chinese philosophy and "I Ching", meditation, symbolism, healing and spiritual science, energy dynamics, breathing and body alignment are taught concurrently with movement study from the 1st Term. Nature imagery, colour, sound and occasionally music are employed in sensitivity, relaxation and attunement training. All areas of study are interrelated as aspects of the One Life, and transmitted in terms of Western cultural reality and everyday life.

Classes are normally $1^1/_2$ hours weekly, and regular attendance, punctuality, commitment and integrity are required. Classes involve both theory and practice – teaching, discussion and movement according to development and interest, particularly in advanced classes.

◆ *Individual guidance* is ensured within the framework of limited size group study and energy.

◆ *A lending library* of wide-ranging books and cassettes are available to students.

◆ *Workshops, talks and group study* sessions are offered regularly or arranged periodically for education, inspiration and social enjoyment.

Intuitive Foot Massage

A subtle, meditative cause-level therapy using flowing touch and aura vibration. *The Certificate Training Course* for small groups involves oil technique, spiritual anatomy, reflexes and attunement. Introductory weekends are available periodically.

Personal Services with Beverley Milne

Spiritual counselling, soul rebuilding, spiritual healing, Intuitive Foot Massage, T'ai-chi, "I Ching", meditation, psychic protection.

Weekly or Monthly Groups

Meditation, spiritual discussion, "I Ching", spiritual talks etc.

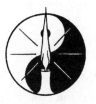

APPENDIX F

Books and Cassettes by Beverley Milne

Available 1994. Published by The Healing School of T'ai-Chi, Melbourne.

Books

◆ TAOISM, THE MYSTICAL WAY OF LAO TZU. An introduction to the origins and influence of Taoism. (1977)

◆ A SURVEY OF CHINESE THOUGHT. A history of philosophical development from animism to "I Ching", Taoism, Confucianism and Buddhism. (1978)

◆ CONSULTING THE "I CHING". Origins, spiritual influences, consultation procedure, and guidance. (1978)

◆ T'AI-CHI SPIRIT AND ESSENCE – A New Vision of a Healing Process. (1994) Revised and expanded. (First published 1979 London)

Monographs

◆ The Heart of T'ai-chi
◆ Tension and the Use of the Mind
◆ Body Alignment
◆ Hints on Food Reform

Sheets for Study

◆ Colour Rays and Correspondences
◆ Aura Colours and Symbolism
◆ Foot Reflexes Chart
◆ Psychic Protection notes
◆ Spectrum of Love   etc.

Colour Plates

◆ 7 Dimensions of Being
◆ Etheric Energy Flows
◆ Affirmation "I AM the Living Spirit"
◆ Affirmation poem

Bookmark

◆ "I AM the Living Spirit"

Cassettes – Lecture/Talk Titles

60 minutes:
◆ Inspiration and the Process of Creative Expression
◆ T'ai-chi and the Spiritual Path
◆ Intuitive Foot Massage
◆ Self-Discipline & Emotional Balance (inc. 10 min. meditation)
◆ T'ai-chi Mirror of the Soul

90 minutes:
◆ "I Ching" and Creative Living
◆ Rhythm, Change and "I Ching"
◆ Spiritual Guidance and Spirit Guides
◆ Psychic Self-Protection 1 and 2
◆ Spirit Guides and the Astral Plane 1 and 2
◆ The Power of Thought
◆ Reincarnation and Karma

120 minutes:
◆ Incarnation, Relationships and Karma
◆ Talking About Colour, Spiritual Teaching and Healing
◆ Soul Development and Guidance
◆ Sexuality and Spirituality
◆ Understanding Masculine and Feminine
◆ Communicating with Spirit   … and others.

For details and price list, please send an S.A.E. to the School.